Practical
Histology
WORKBOOK

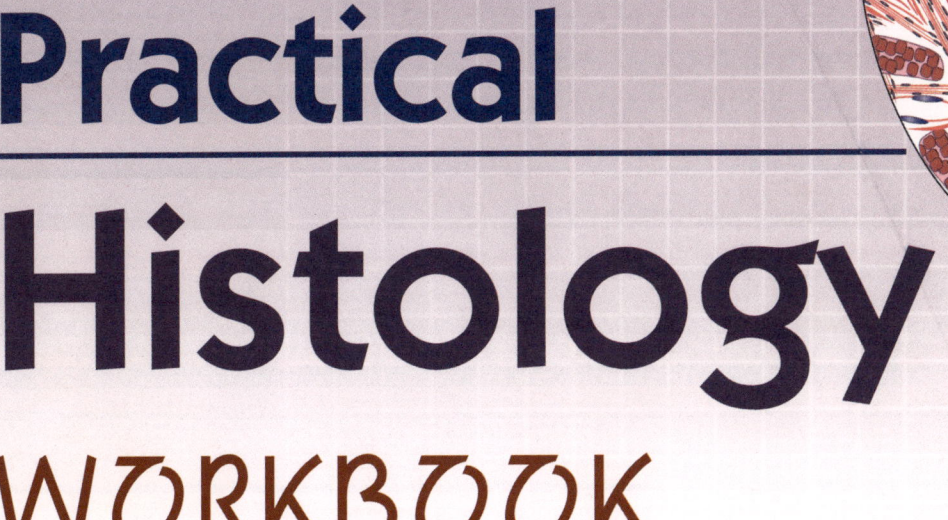

Revised Second Edition

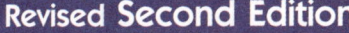

Student's Name _____

Roll No. _____   Year/Session _____

University Roll No. _____   Name of the Course _____

Name of the Institution _____

This is to certify that this is a bonafide practical work done by _____ *during the year 20____ – 20____. His/her work is complete | incomplete | excellent | satisfactory | good | fair.*

_____   _____

Signature of Staff in-charge   Signature of Professor & HoD

Submitted for University Examination in the year _____

Examiners: _____   _____

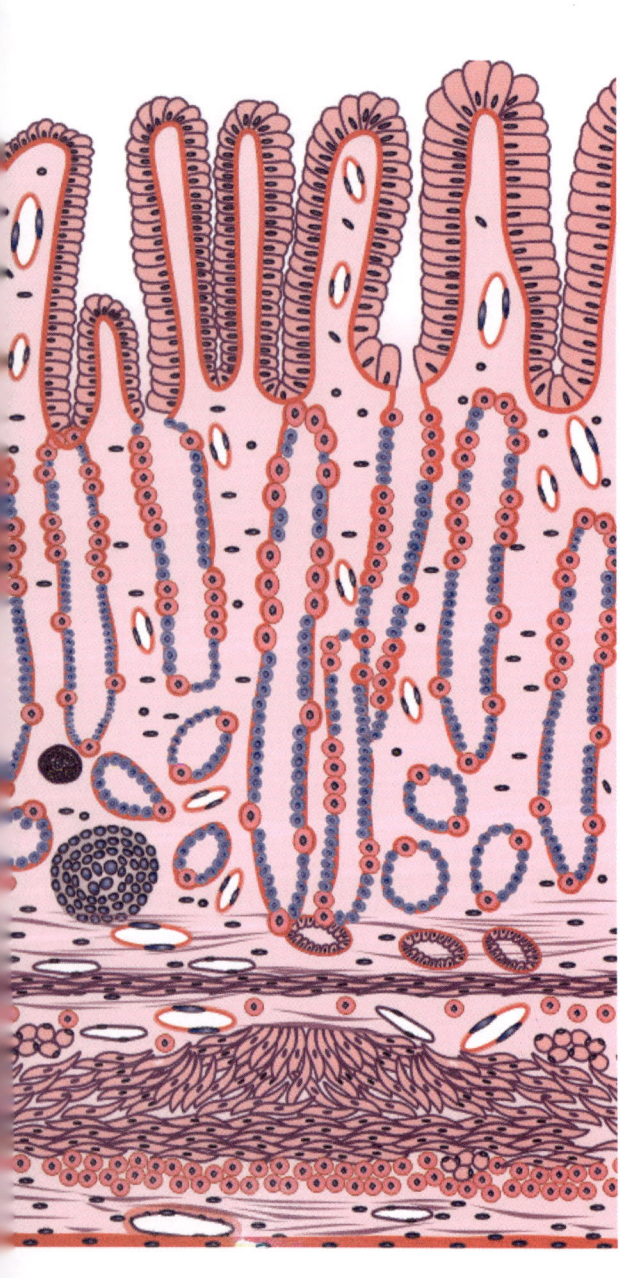

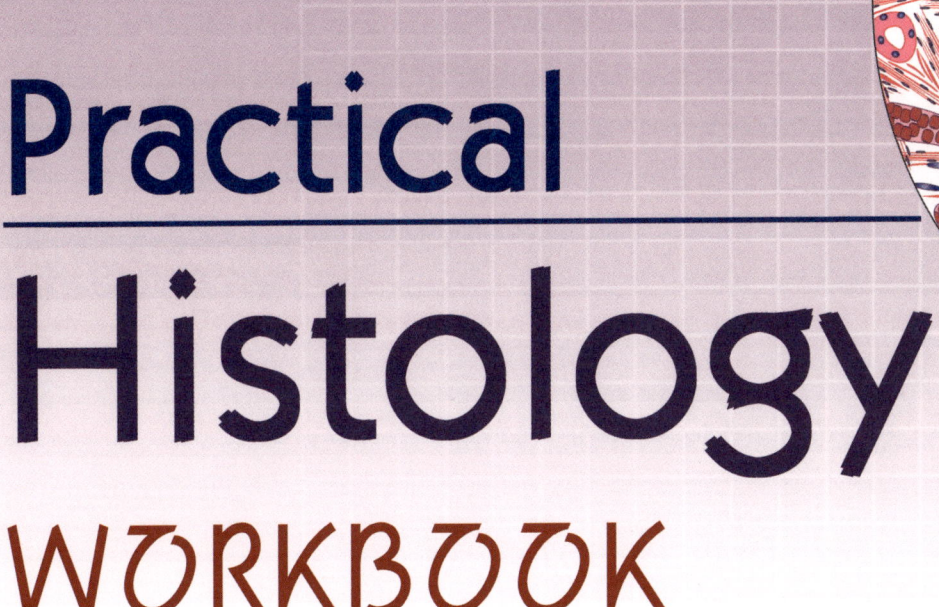

Practical
Histology
WORKBOOK

Revised Second Edition

Krishna Garg

MBBS MS PhD FIMSA FIAMS FAMS, FASI

ex-Professor and Head
Department of Anatomy
Lady Hardinge Medical College
New Delhi

Shilpa Garg

MBBS MD

Wilmington Veterans Affair Hospital
Delaware, USA

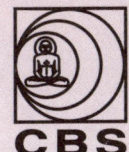
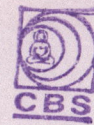

CBS Publishers & Distributors Pvt Ltd

New Delhi • Bengaluru • Chennai • Kochi • Kolkata • Mumbai
Hyderabad • Jharkhand • Nagpur • Patna • Pune • Uttarakhand

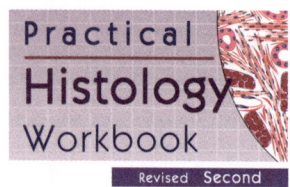

ISBN: 978-93-85915-74-1

Revised Second Edition: 2017

Reprint: 2018

Second Edition: 2016

First Edition: 2014

Published by Satish Kumar Jain and produced by Varun Jain for

CBS Publishers & Distributors Pvt Ltd

4819/XI Prahlad Street, 24 Ansari Road, Daryaganj, New Delhi 110 002, India.
Ph: 23289259, 23266861, 23266867 Website: www.cbspd.com
Fax: 011-23243014   e-mail: delhi@cbspd.com; cbspubs@airtelmail.in.
Corporate Office: 204 FIE, Industrial Area, Patparganj, Delhi 110 092

Ph: 4934 4934   Fax: 4934 4935   e-mail: publishing@cbspd.com; publicity@cbspd.com

Branches

- **Bengaluru:** Seema House 2975, 17th Cross, K.R. Road,
  Banasankari 2nd Stage, Bengaluru 560 070, Karnataka
  Ph: +91-80-26771678/79   Fax: +91-80-26771680   e-mail: bangalore@cbspd.com
- **Chennai:** 7, Subbaraya Street, Shenoy Nagar, Chennai 600 030, Tamil Nadu
  Ph: +91-44-26680620, 26681266   Fax: +91-44-42032115   e-mail: chennai@cbspd.com
- **Kochi:** Ashana House, No. 39/1904, AM Thomas Road, Valanjambalam,
  Ernakulam 682 016, Kochi, Kerala
  Ph: +91-484-4059061-65   Fax: +91-484-4059065   e-mail: kochi@cbspd.com
- **Kolkata:** 6/B, Ground Floor, Rameswar Shaw Road, Kolkata-700 014, West Bengal
  Ph: +91-33-22891126, 22891127, 22891128   e-mail: kolkata@cbspd.com
- **Mumbai:** 83-C, Dr E Moses Road, Worli, Mumbai-400018, Maharashtra
  Ph: +91-22-24902340/41   Fax: +91-22-24902342   e-mail: mumbai@cbspd.com

Representatives

| ï Hyderabad | 0-9885175004 | ï Jharkhand | 0-9811541605 | ï Nagpur | 0-9021734563 |
| ï Patna | 0-9334159340 | ï Pune | 0-9623451994 | ï Uttarakhand | 0-9716462459 |

Printed at Goyal Offset, Delhi, India

Preface to the Second Edition

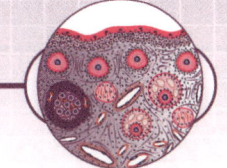

It is our pleasure to acknowledge the fact that after successful launching of the first edition of **Practical Histology** Workbook, we are now presenting the second edition of the Workbook with a large number of features that will make this an extremely useful book for the students. We are sure that the teachers will equally appreciate this publication as it will greatly help them in organising practical class work.

All the diagrams of histology have now been rendered in full color to help the student understand the microscopic structures, identify the tissues, and draw the illustrations in the practical class with clarity and ease. Cell structures have been further improved to bring in anatomic clarity; fresh labelling has been introduced. The brief descriptions have been thoroughly revised and modified to eliminate any conceptual errors.

Based on the feedback from a large number of the students and the teachers who have used the workbook, many of the diagrams have been improved substantially. We hope that this edition will serve the students and the teachers in a manner that will lend clarity, ease, understanding and convenience in its usage.

Thanks to Dr (Prof) Sunanda Raina and her team from Medical College, Jammu, for their valuable suggestion. We are indebted to Dr (Prof) Anupama Mahajan of SGRD Medical College, Amritsar, for supporting this workbook.

Suggestions for further improvement in text and graphics may please be sent at
e-mail: *dr.krishnagarg@gmail.com.*

Krishna Garg
Shilpa Garg

Preface to the First Edition

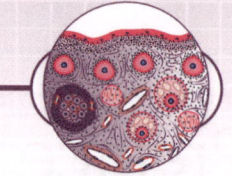

Practical Histology *Workbook* would make practicals easy. Introduction to the chapter and a few points about the tissue, including its black and white diagram, is provided on the left-hand side page. The right-hand side page represents the student's page. The histology of tissue, as seen through the microscope, is to be drawn using colours representing haematoxylin and eosin stains. The three key points of identification of each figure are to be written in the space provided. Stains which colour the slides accentuate the subtle differences between normal and abnormal cells and tissues. Thus these are vital for correct diagnosis and proper treatment.

Key to identification of histological slides given in Chapter 20 provides a quick way towards achieving the goal.

Lack of space for any additional text or diagram has been compensated by blank space labelled 'Notes' with a few chapters and two blank pages labelled 'Additional figures/notes' at the end of some chapters.

Histology teaches the microscopic structure of normal tissues so that any abnormality occurring due to disease process may be diagnosed during the later period of studies and practice.

We are indebted to Dr Medha Joshi for always lending a helping hand. We are extremely thankful to Mr SK Jain, CMD; Mr YN Arjuna, Senior Vice-President—Publishing, Editorial and Promotion; Ms Ritu Chawla, AGM–Production; and other supporting staff of CBSP&D, for their help and guidance in completing this work.

Krishna Garg

Shilpa Garg

Contents

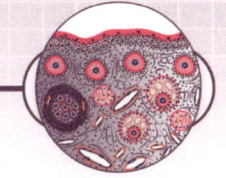

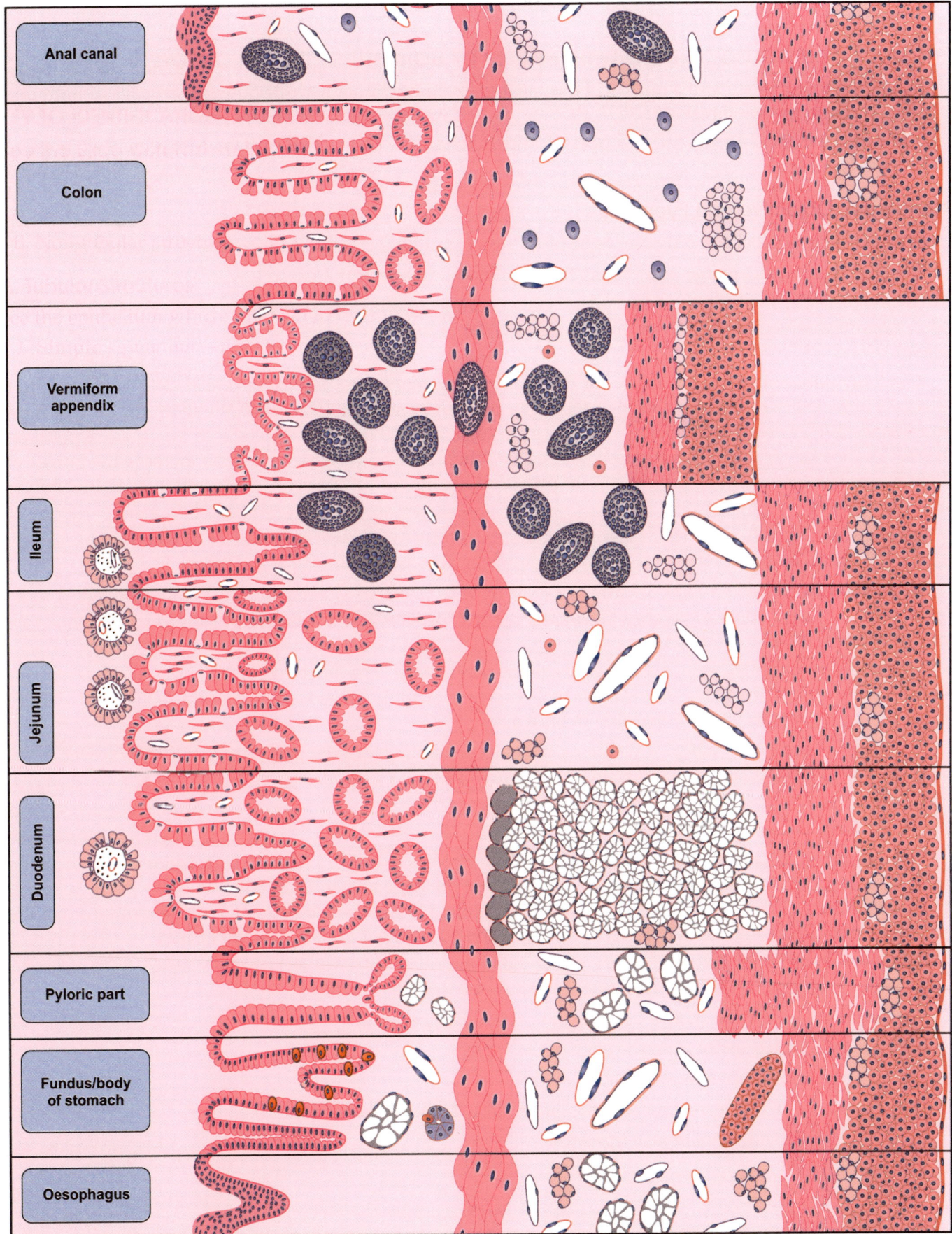

Anal canal

Colon

Vermiform appendix

Ileum

Jejunum

Duodenum

Pyloric part

Fundus/body of stomach

Oesophagus

1. Microscope

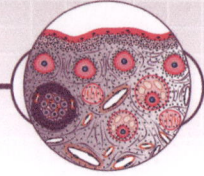

THE STUDY OF HISTOLOGY IS DONE WITH THE HELP OF LIGHT/STUDENT'S MICROSCOPE

The light microscope/student's microscope is used to examine the stained specimens by means of light that courses through the specimen.

Light microscope is composed of optical and mechanical parts. The optical components comprise 3 systems of lenses:

Condenser, Objective and Eyepiece

The condenser lens collects and focuses light, emitting a cone of light that illuminates the tissues to be observed.

The objective lenses enlarge and project the illuminated image of the tissue towards the eyepiece.

The eyepiece further magnifies the image received and projects it to the viewer/photographic plate. The total magnification is obtained by multiplying the power of the objective lens with that of the ocular/eyepiece lens.

Resolving power: It is critical factor for obtaining ideal image. The resolving power (RP) is the smallest distance between two particles at which these can be seen as separate objects. The maximum RP of a light microscope is 0.2 μm. This RP can be magnified up to 1000–1500 times. The details of the tissue depend on the RP of the microscope. Magnification is of value when RP is high. Video cameras increase the power of light microscope. Usually two objectives are provided in student's microscopes 10X and 40X, or low power and high power.

Eyepiece lens usually have 10X. Magnification obtained by low power objective is 10 when multiplied by 10X = 100 times. Magnification obtained by high power objective is 40 × 10 = 400 times.

Mechanical parts: Microscope consists of a joint or base which is 'U' shaped. The base is connected to an 'arm'. At the upper end of arm is the tube for supporting the lenses. The tube can be moved up and down by coarse and fine adjustment knobs.

At the lower end of the arm is fastened a square plate/stage. The stage has an opening in the centre for light to pass through the tissue. The stage is further provided with 2 clips to keep the slide stationary or there is movable mechanism to move the slide in both axes.

At the lower end of the tube is a revolving nosepiece with 2 objectives, low power and high power.

A mirror is placed below the condenser lens directs the light from the lamp/sun towards the specimen. The mirror has two surfaces, one plane and other concave. The plane mirror is used with the condenser and concave mirror is used when condenser is not in use.

Viewing the slide: Place lamp 6 inches away from the microscope. Use substage condenser and plane mirror. Adjust mirror so get uniform light. Put the slide on stage and strap it with clips. Lower the tube, till the lower power objective is about 5 mm above the slide. Use coarse adjustment knob to gently move the tube upwards till the specimen is viewed. Now use fire adjustment knob to see the details.

For viewing with high power objective, rotate the high power objective on nosepiece above the tissue till a click sound is obtained. Use fine adjustment knob to see greater details.

Precautions: Microscope should be held and carried by both hands.

It should be 6 inches away from the edge of the table.

The arm should be kept straight or titled slightly only.

The microscope to be cleaned before use with a silky cloth and never a handkerchief.

Cover slip of the slide should face upwards.

Microscope

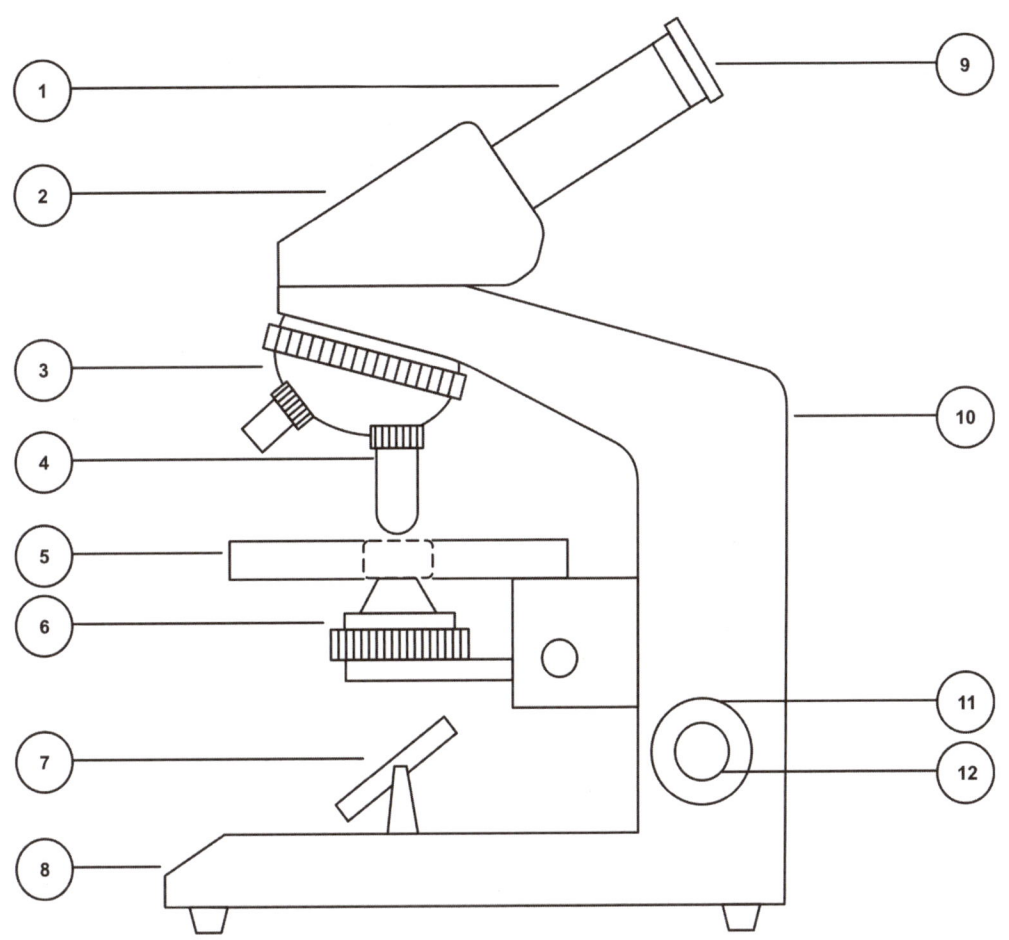

Label the diagram

1. _____   2. _____

3. _____   4. _____

5. _____   6. _____

7. _____   8. _____

9. _____   10. _____

11. _____   12. _____

2. Epithelium

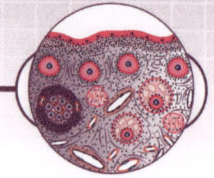

Histology is the microscopic study of various tissues of the body. A tissue is made up of groups of cells performing the same function. The cell is the basic structural unit of the body. The cell consists of a cell membrane enclosing the cytoplasm with a nucleus usually in the centre.

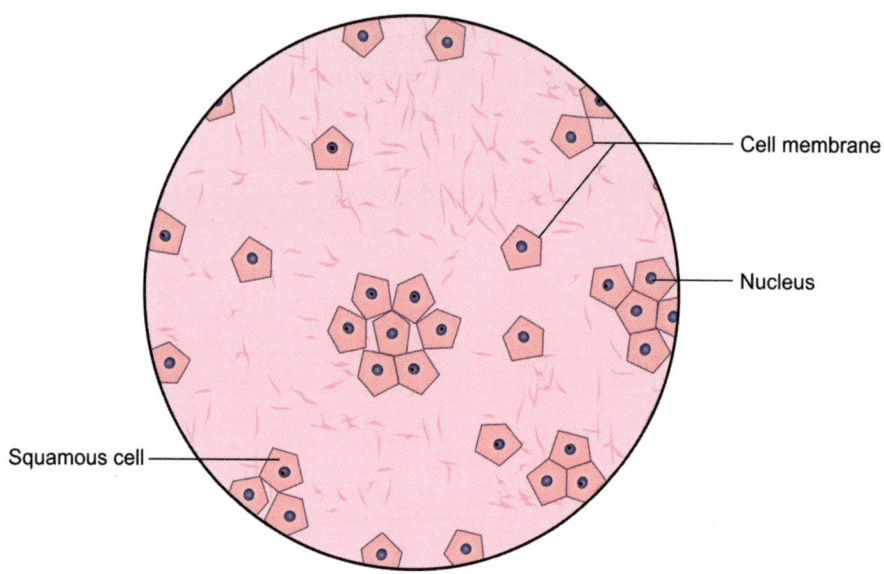

Desquamated squamous cells—cheek mucosa

FUNCTIONS OF EPITHELIAL TISSUE/EPITHELIUM

a. *Protective*: The stratified squamous keratinised epithelium of skin offers mechanical protection including conservation of moisture.

b. *Secretory*: _____

c. *Absorptive*: _____

_____

d. *Excretory*: _____

_____

e. *Sensory*: _____

_____

Characters of Epithelium

_____

_____

_____

_____

_____

_____

Desquamated Squamous Cells

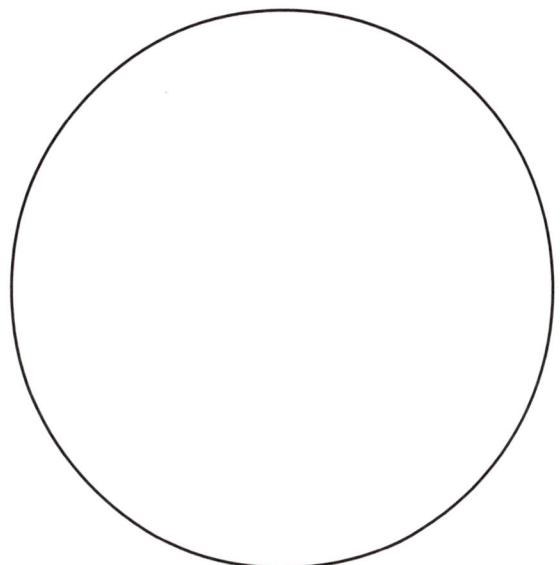

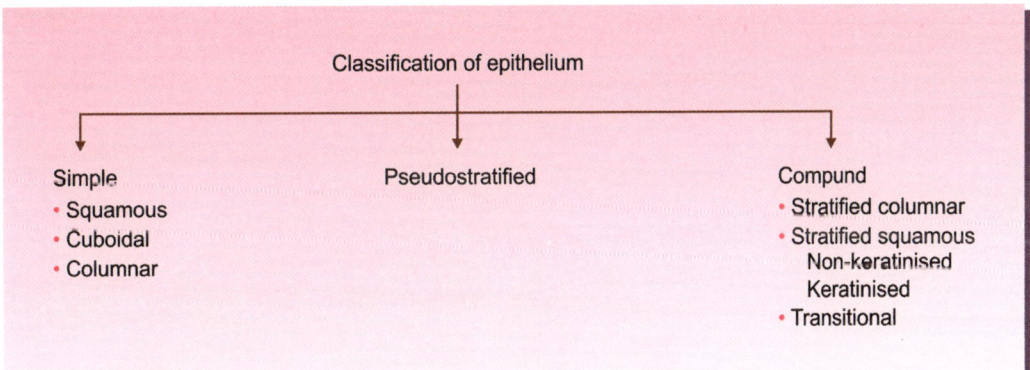

Facts
to
Remember

Classification of epithelium

Simple
• Squamous
• Cuboidal
• Columnar

Pseudostratified

Compund
• Stratified columnar
• Stratified squamous
  Non-keratinised
  Keratinised
• Transitional

Notes

SIMPLE EPITHELIUM

It can be of the following types:

a. *Squamous (scale like) or pavement epithelium,* e.g. alveoli of lungs, endothelium of blood vessels and mesothelium of serous membranes. The epithelium in sections is seen to consist of a single layer of thin cells with flattened nuclei.

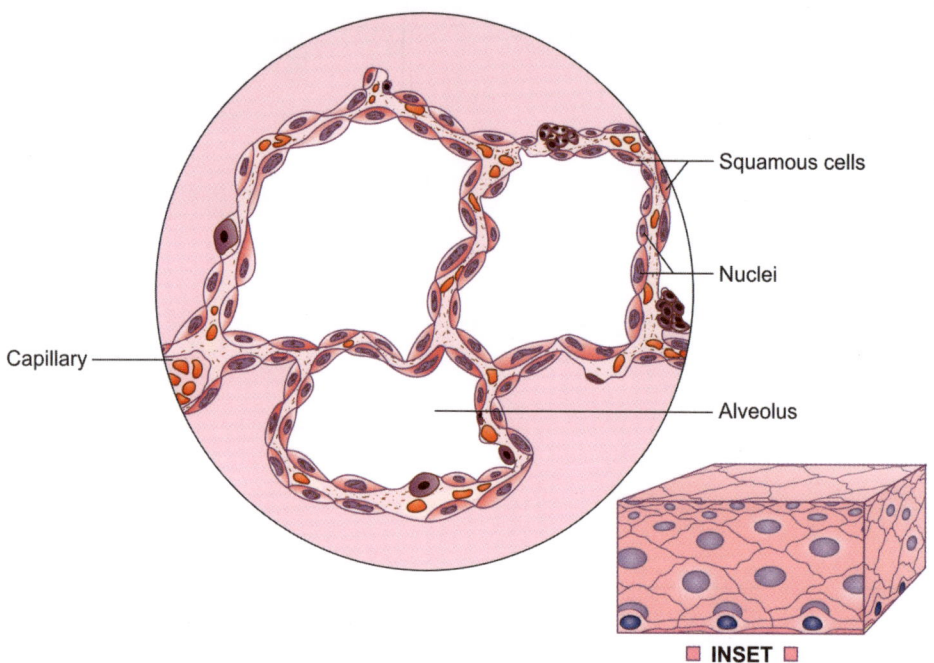

Alveoli of lungs. Stain: Haematoxylin-eosin, 400X

b. *Cuboidal epithelium:* Thyroid gland acini during resting phase, small ducts of the glands. The cells have equal width and height with the round central nuclei.

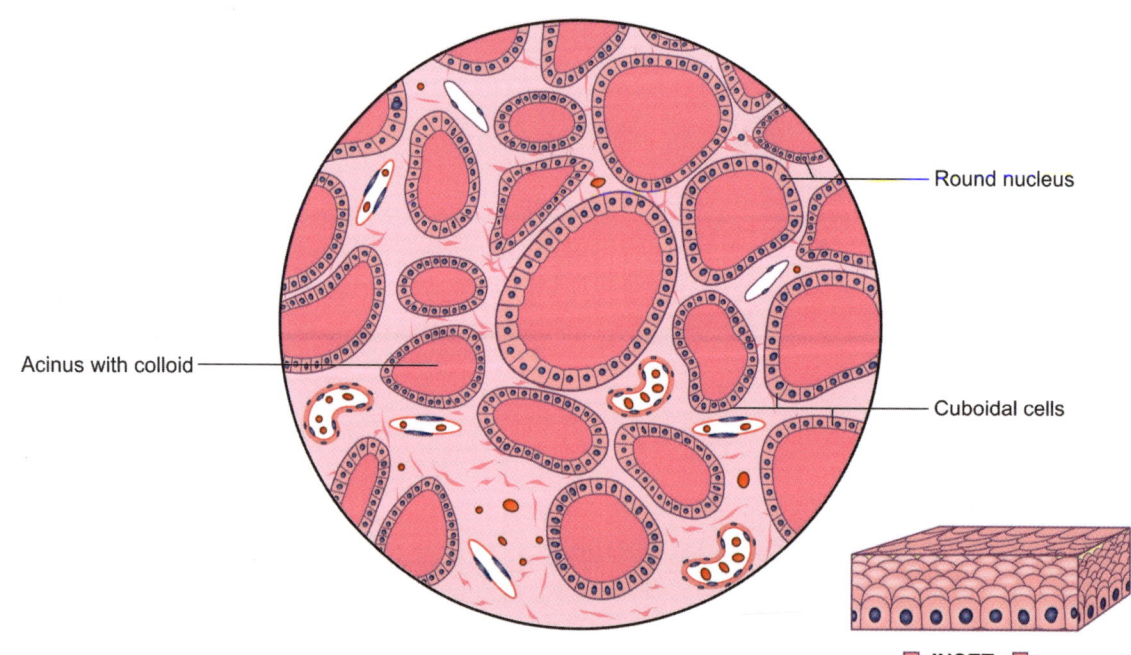

Thyroid gland. Stain: Haematoxylin-eosin, 100X

Squamous Epithelium

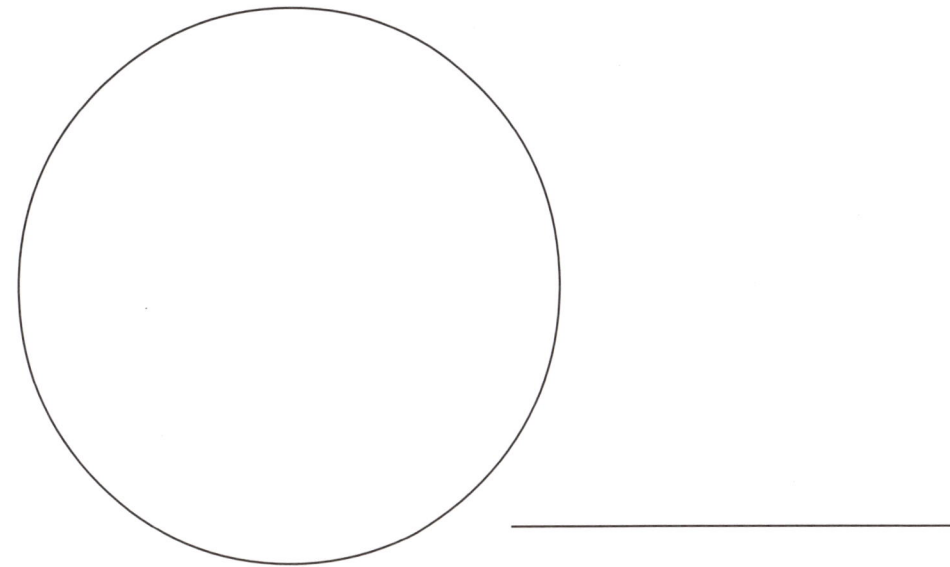

_____

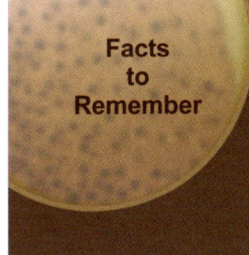

**Facts
to
Remember**

_____

_____

_____

_____

Cuboidal Epithelium

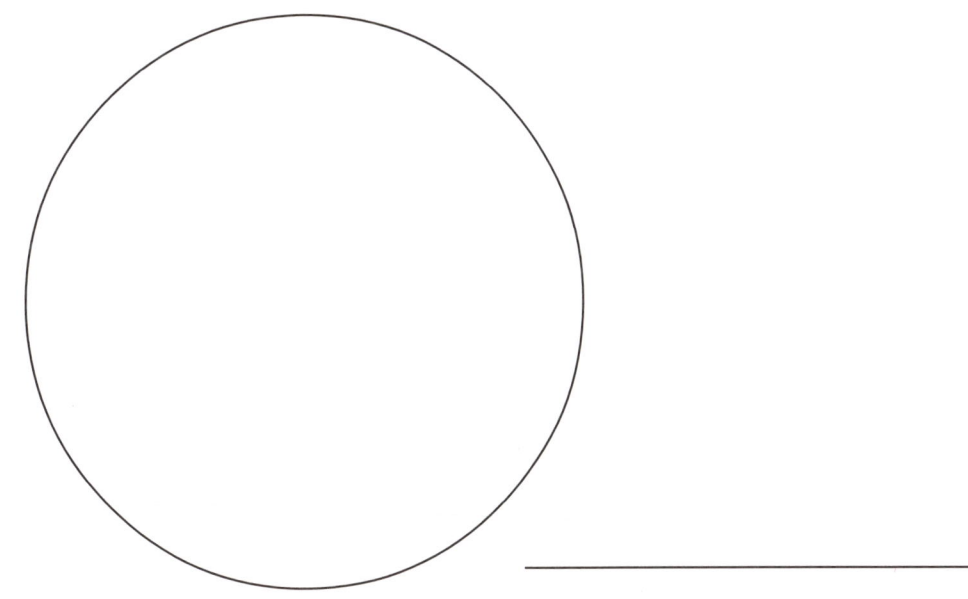

_____

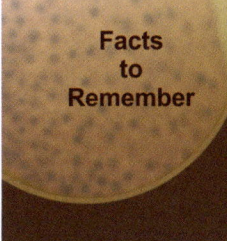

**Facts
to
Remember**

_____

_____

_____

c. *Columnar epithelium:* The cells are almost three times taller than their width. Nucleus is basal and oval in shape seen in. Its modifications are as follows.

i. *Simple columnar epithelium:* _____

_____

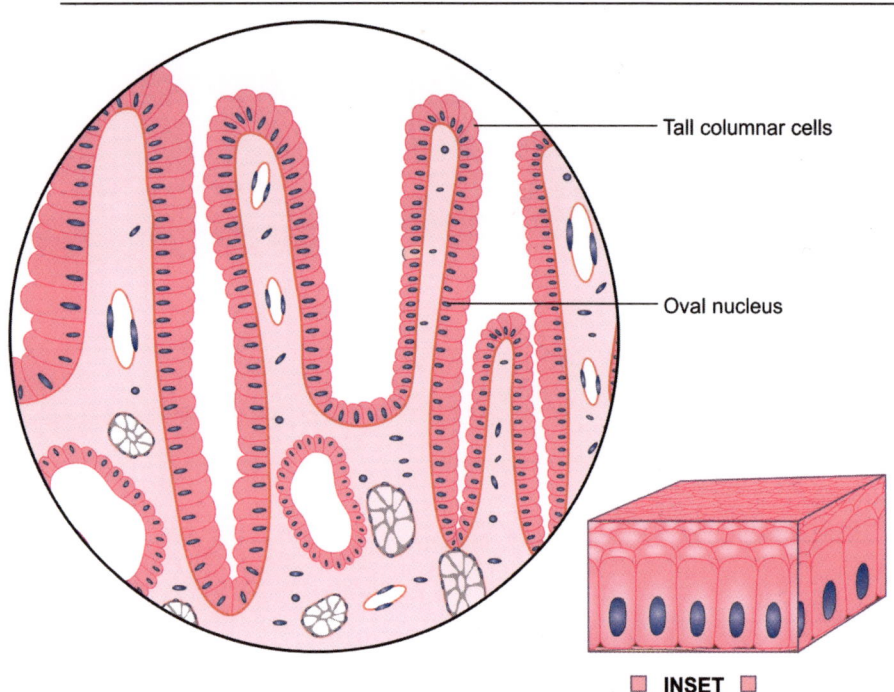

Stomach. Stain: Haematoxylin-eosin, 400X

ii. *Columnar cells with microvilli or brush border:* _____

_____

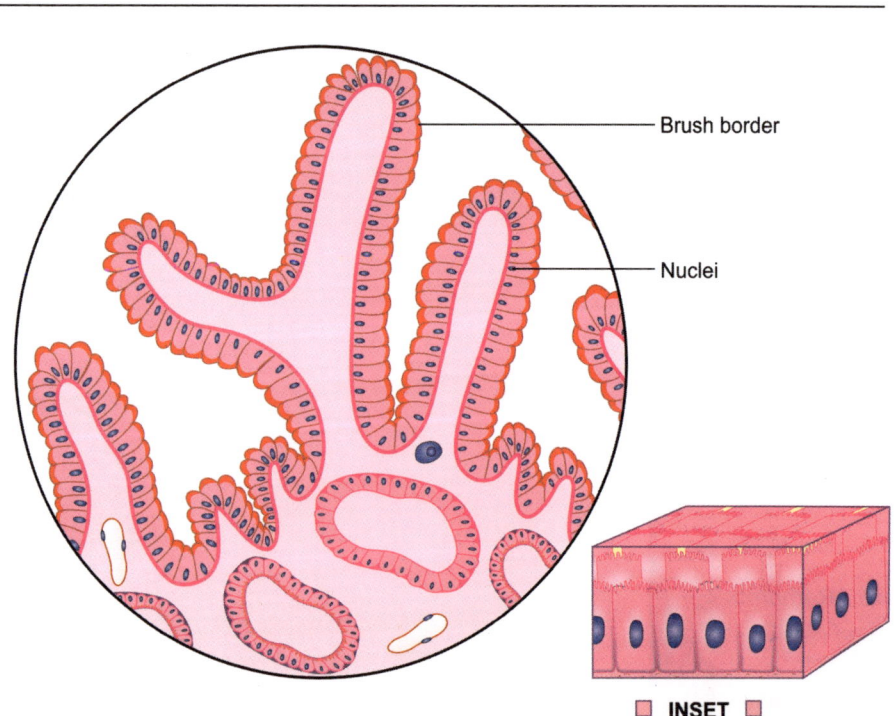

Gall bladder. Stain: Haematoxylin-eosin, 400X

Simple Columnar Epithelium

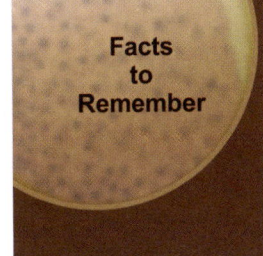

Facts to Remember

_____

_____

_____

Columnar Epithelium with Brush Border

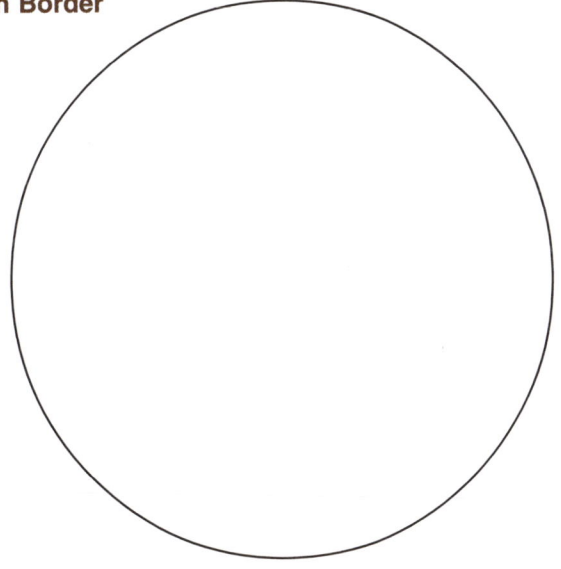

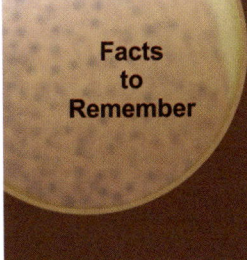

Facts to Remember

_____

_____

_____

iii. *Ciliated columnar epithelium:* _____

_____

_____

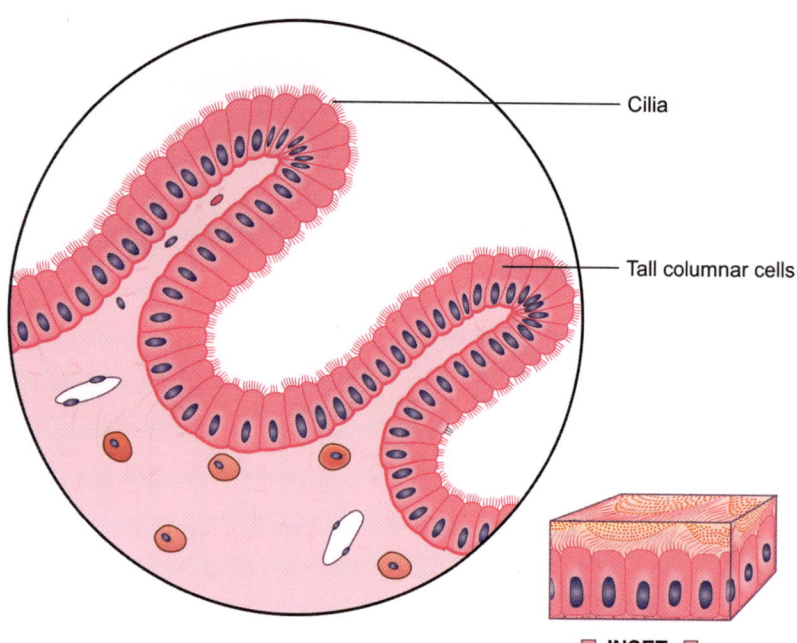

Cilia

Tall columnar cells

INSET

Fallopian tube. Stain: Haematoxylin-eosin, 400X

iv. *Goblet cells:* _____

_____

_____

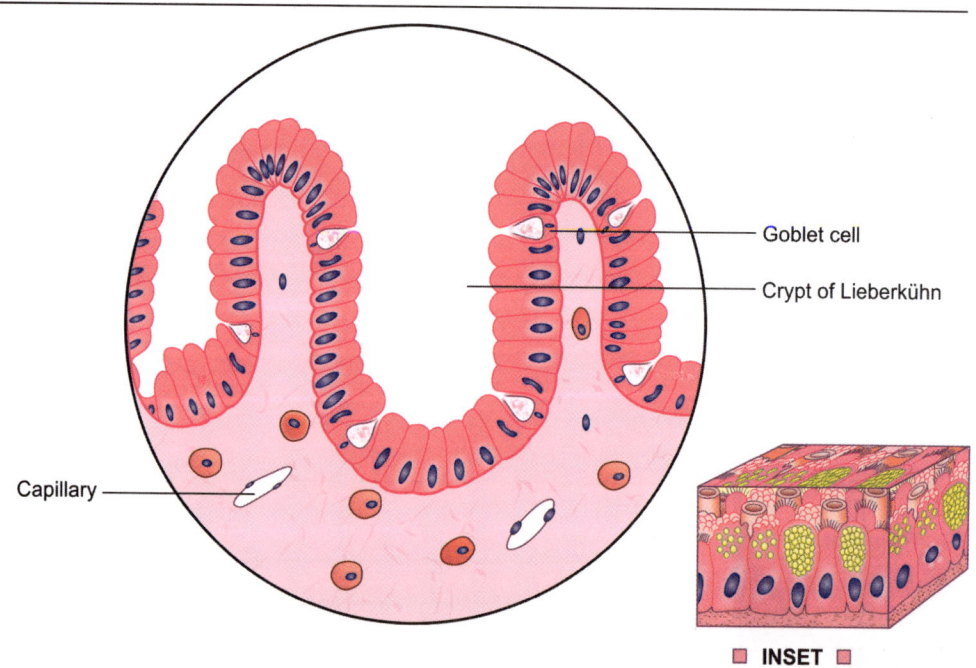

Goblet cell

Crypt of Lieberkühn

Capillary

INSET

Colon. Stain: Haematoxylin-eosin, 400X

Ciliated Columnar Epithelium

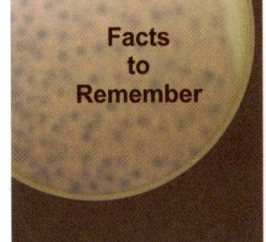

Facts
to
Remember

_____

_____

_____

Goblet Cells

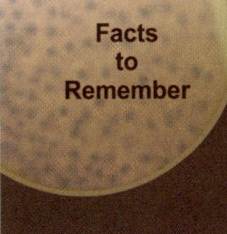

Facts
to
Remember

_____

_____

_____

PSEUDOSTRATIFIED EPITHELIUM

_____

_____

_____

_____

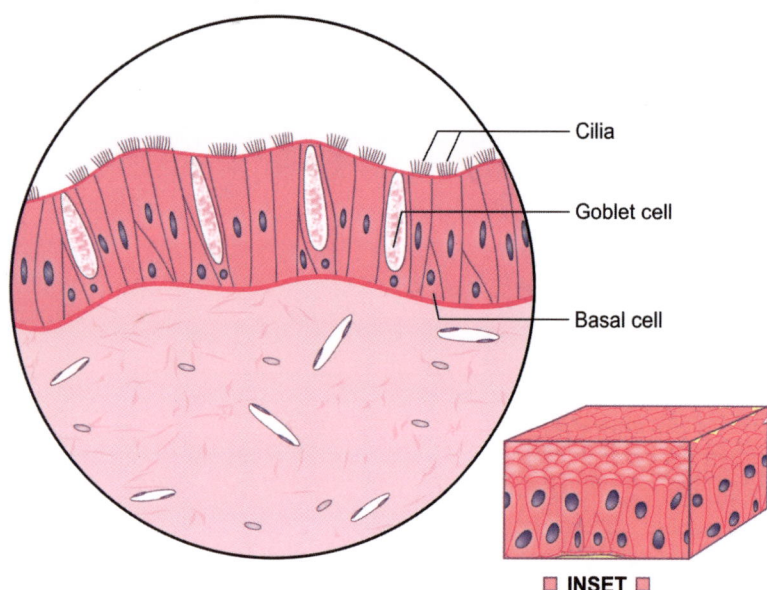

Trachea. Stain: Haematoxylin-eosin, 400X

COMPOUND EPITHELIUM

a. Stratified columnar epithelium: _____

_____

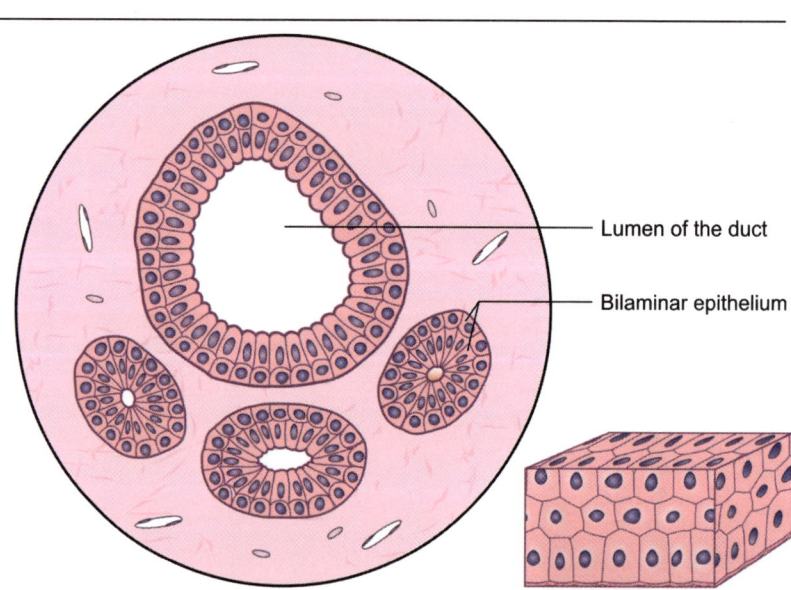

Large duct. Stain: Haematoxylin-eosin, 400X

Pseudostratified Columnar Ciliated Epithelium

**Facts
to
Remember**

_____

_____

_____

Stratified Columnar Epithelium

**Facts
to
Remember**

_____

_____

_____

b. *Stratified squamous non-keratinised type:* Example is oesophagus; oral cavity, vagina. The cells occur in three layers or zones as follows:

i. _____

ii. _____

iii. _____

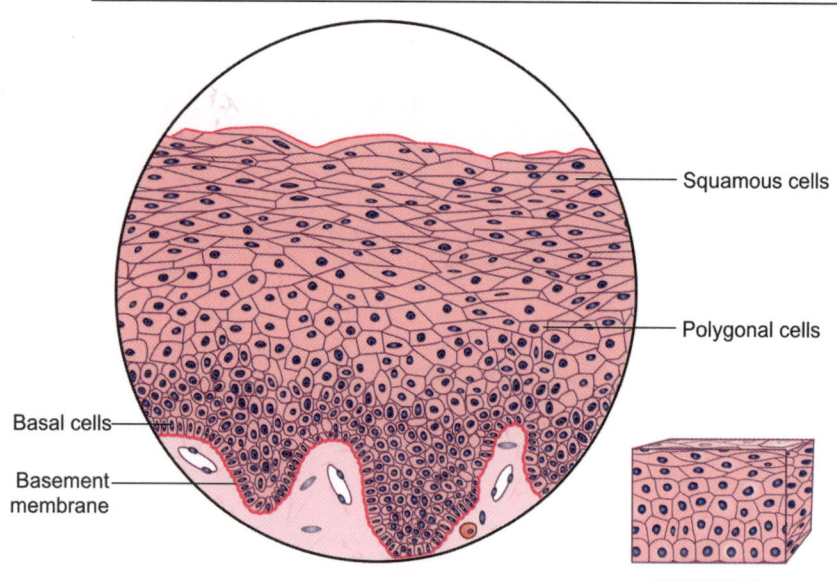

Basal cells

Basement membrane

Squamous cells

Polygonal cells

INSET

Oesophagus. Stain: Haematoxylin-eosin, 400X

c. *Stratified squamous keratinised epithelium*

Seen in skin. The layers or zones are as follows:

i. *Stratum basale or stratum germinativum:* _____

ii. *Stratum spinosum:* _____

iii. *Stratum granulosum:* _____

iv. *Stratum lucidum:* _____

v. *Stratum corneum:* _____

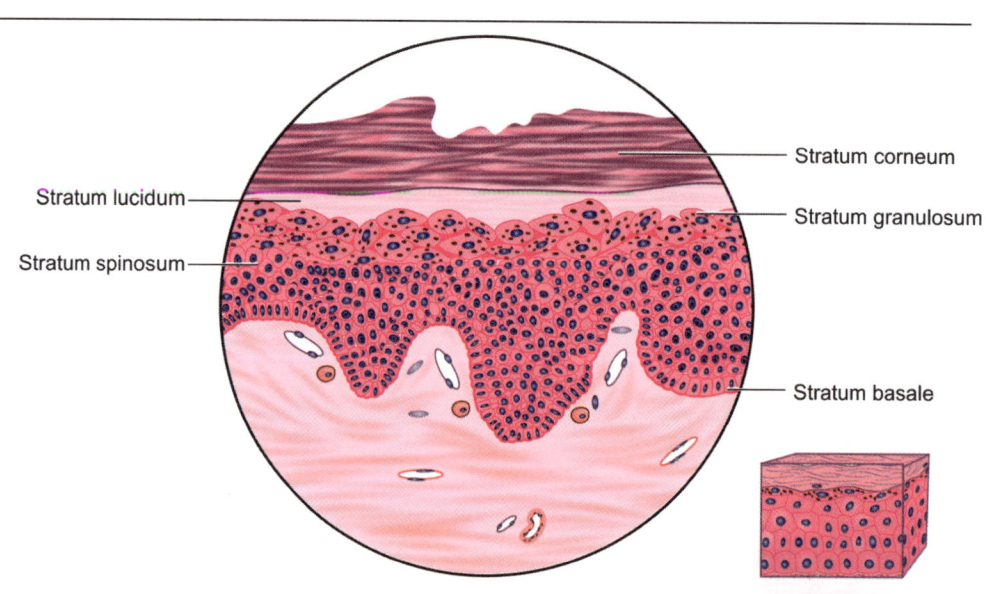

Stratum lucidum

Stratum spinosum

Stratum corneum

Stratum granulosum

Stratum basale

INSET

Skin. Stain: Haematoxylin-eosin, 400X

Stratified Squamous Non-keratinised Epithelium

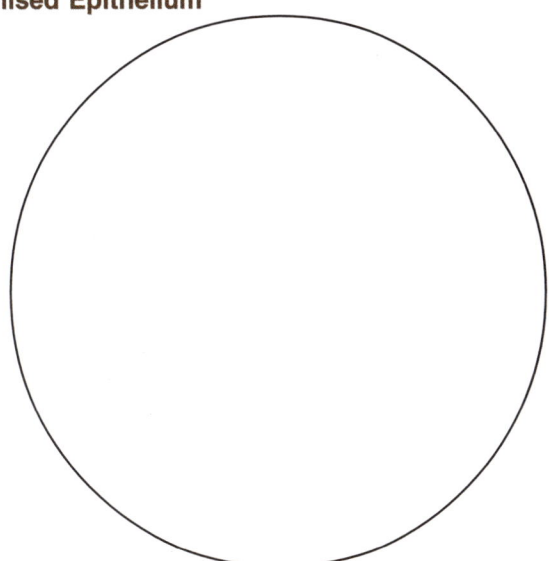

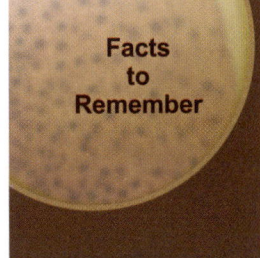

**Facts
to
Remember**

_____

_____

_____

Stratified Squamous Keratinised Epithelium

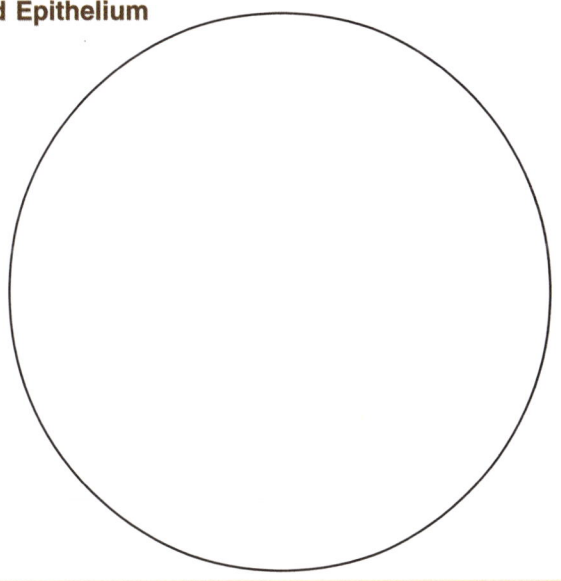

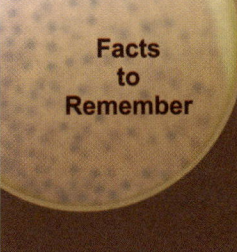

**Facts
to
Remember**

_____

_____

_____

d. *Transitional epithelium*

_____

_____

_____

_____

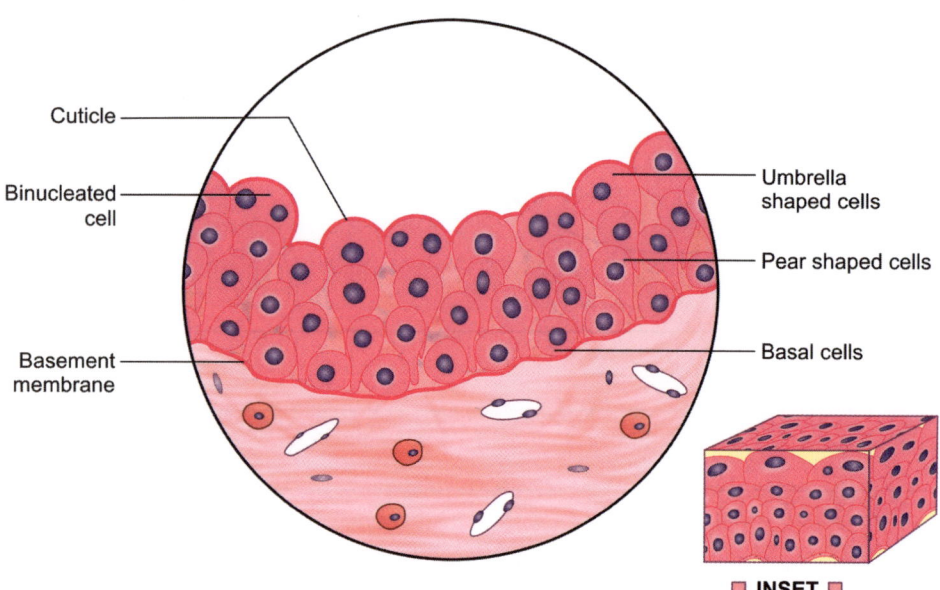

Ureter. Stain: Haematoxylin-eosin, 400X

Transitional Epithelium

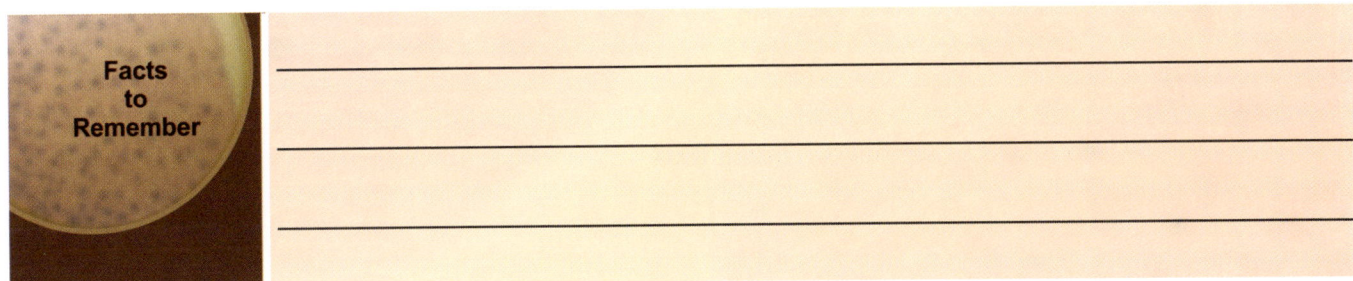

Facts
to
Remember

Notes

3. Connective Tissue

As the name suggests, the connective tissue binds and weaves through diverse tissues of the body. Connective tissue is composed of cells, fibres and ground substance.

The cells may be:

1. Fixed, e.g. fibroblast cells, adipose/fat cells, mesenchymal cells and pigment cell; or
2. Wandering, e.g. macrophages/histiocyte cell, plasma cell, mast cell and other white blood cells.

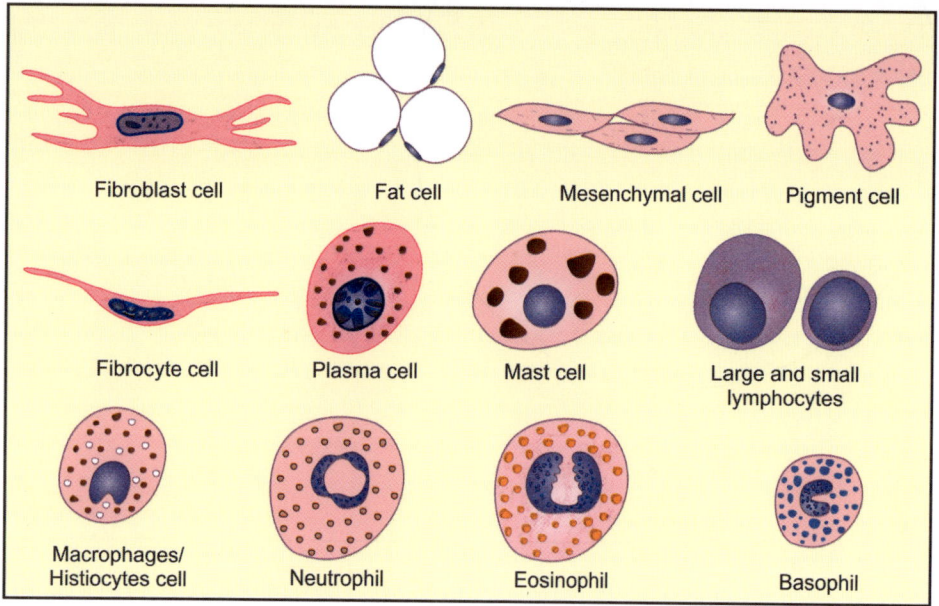

Various cells of connective tissue, 400X

Fibres are of three types:

1. _____
2. _____
3. _____

Collagen fibres

Reticular fibres

Elastic fibres

Various fibres of connective tissue, 100X

Ground Substance

The formed elements of connective tissue, e.g. cells and fibres are embedded in the ground substance. Intercellular substance is the term used for combination of ground substance and fibres. Ground substance is comprised of water, carbohydrate and glycoproteins.

Connective Tissue Cells

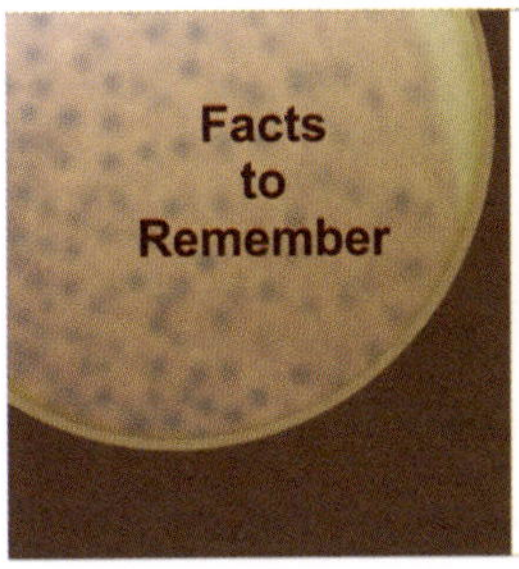

**Facts
to
Remember**

Fibres

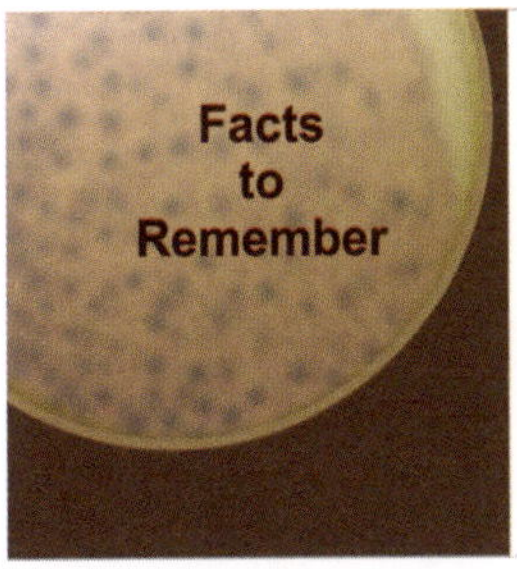

**Facts
to
Remember**

Loose Connective Tissue

1. *Areolar tissue*

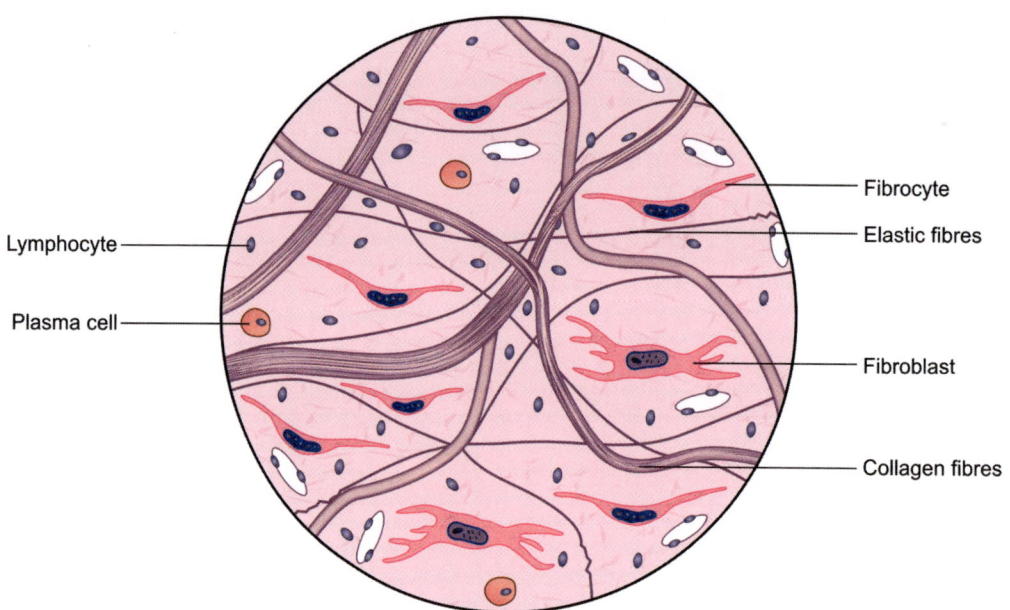

Lymphocyte

Plasma cell

Fibrocyte

Elastic fibres

Fibroblast

Collagen fibres

Superficial fascia. Stain: Haematoxylin-eosin, 100X

2. *Adipose tissue*

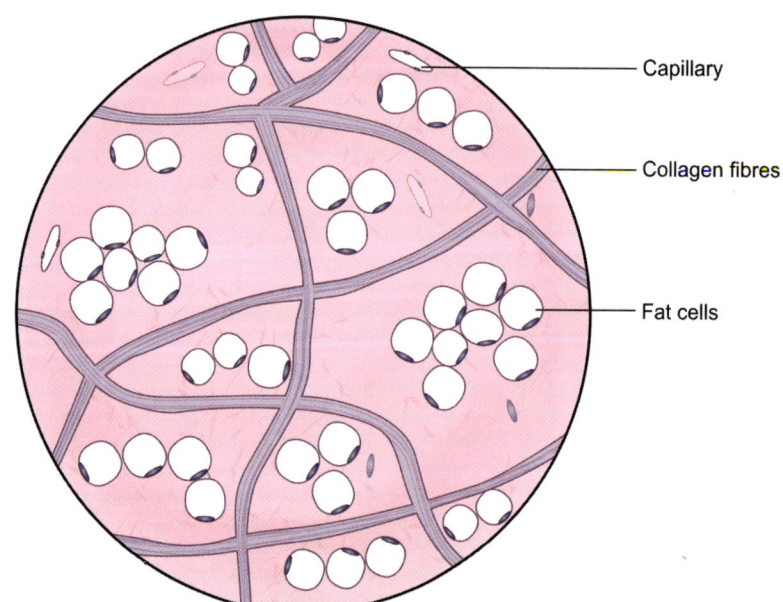

Capillary

Collagen fibres

Fat cells

Mesentery. Stain: Haematoxylin-eosin, 100X

Areolar Tissue

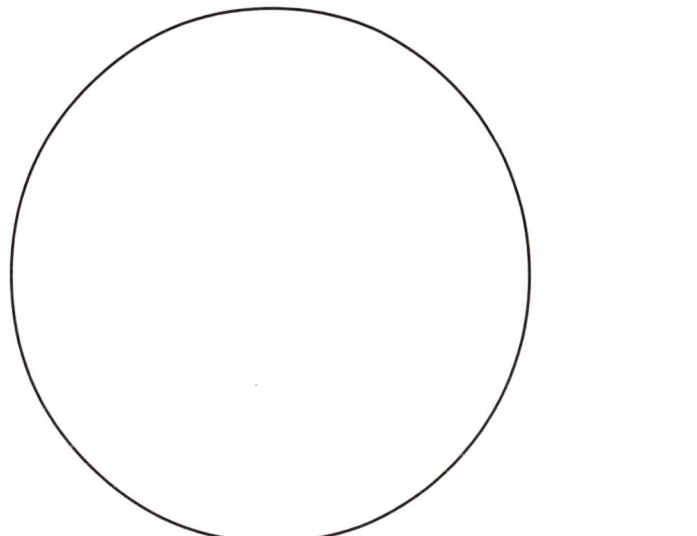

_____

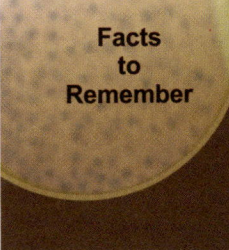

Facts to Remember

_____

_____

_____

Adipose Tissue

_____

Facts to Remember

_____

_____

_____

3. *Reticular tissue* _____

_____

_____

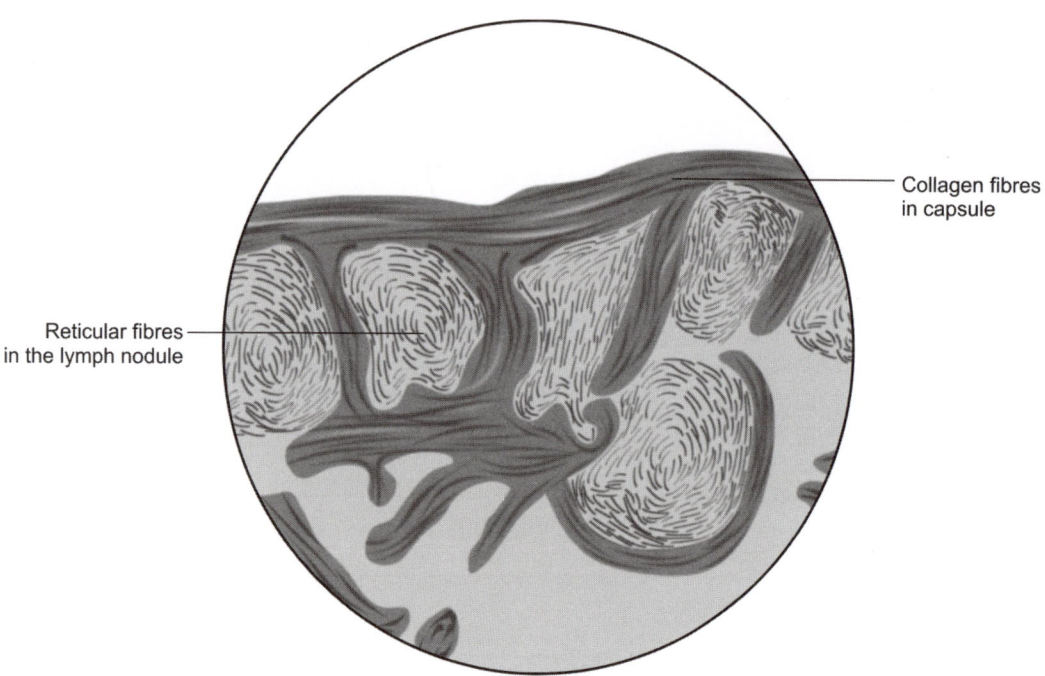

Lymph node. Stain: Reticulin stain, 100X

4. *Myxomatous tissue* _____

_____

_____

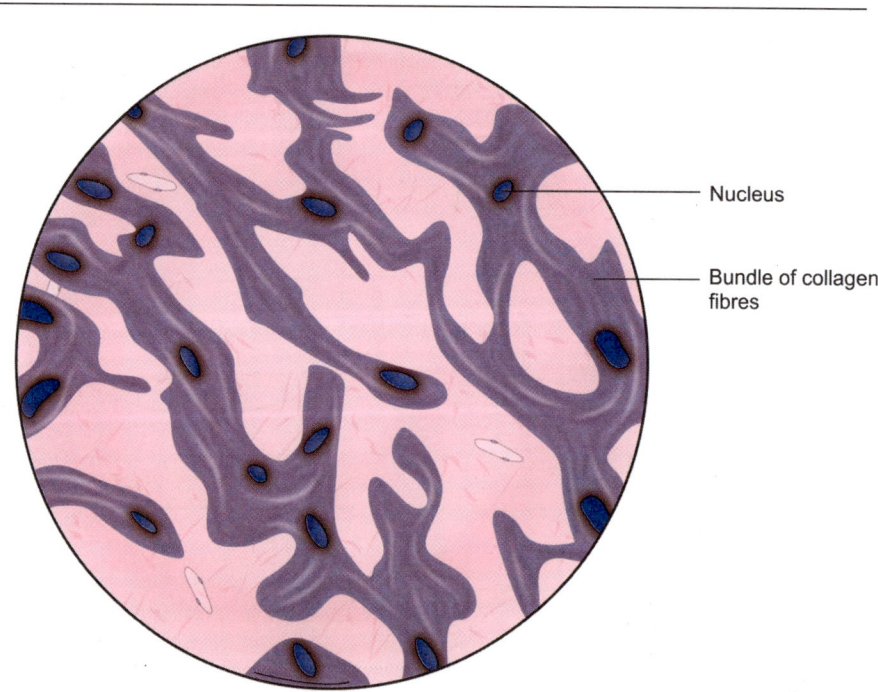

Umbilical cord. Stain: Haematoxylin-eosin, 100X

Reticular Tissue

Facts to Remember

_____

_____

_____

_____

Myxomatous Tissue

Facts to Remember

_____

_____

_____

_____

DENSE CONNECTIVE TISSUE

Ordinary irregular dense connective tissue is seen in the dermis of skin which comprises collagen fibres situated in outer papillary layer and inner reticular layers.

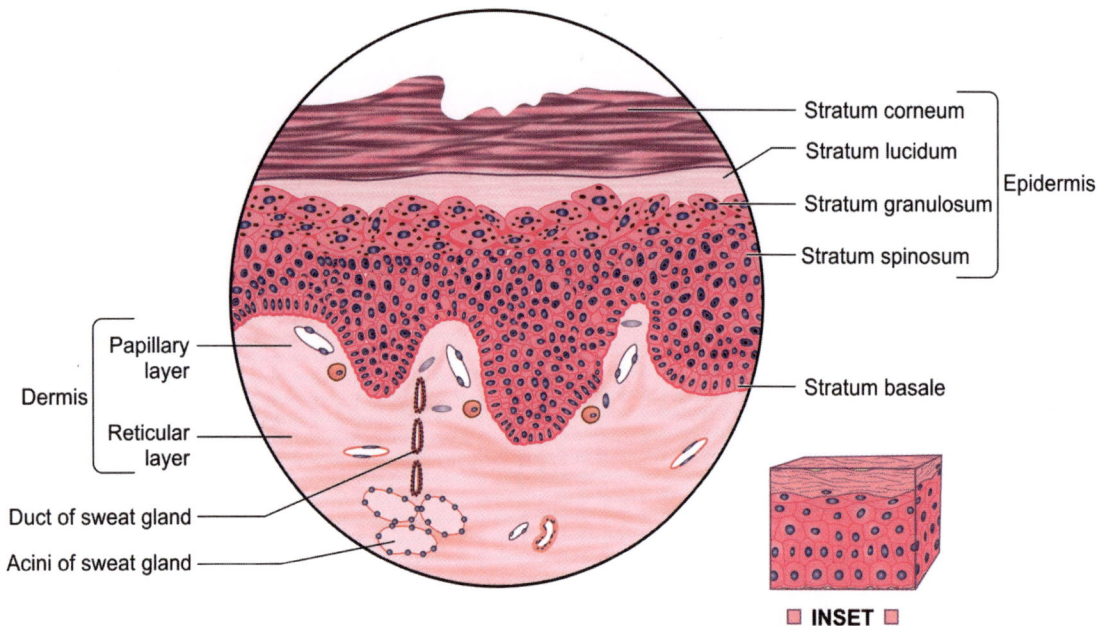

Dermis of skin. Stain: Haematoxylin-eosin, 100X

Ordinary regular dense connective tissue: The collagen fibres are arranged in closely packed bundles in regular parallel manner with fibroblast nuclei which get pressed due to pressure of fibres. This type of tissue is seen in tendons of the muscles. Tendons are easily visible on the dorsum of hands and feet.

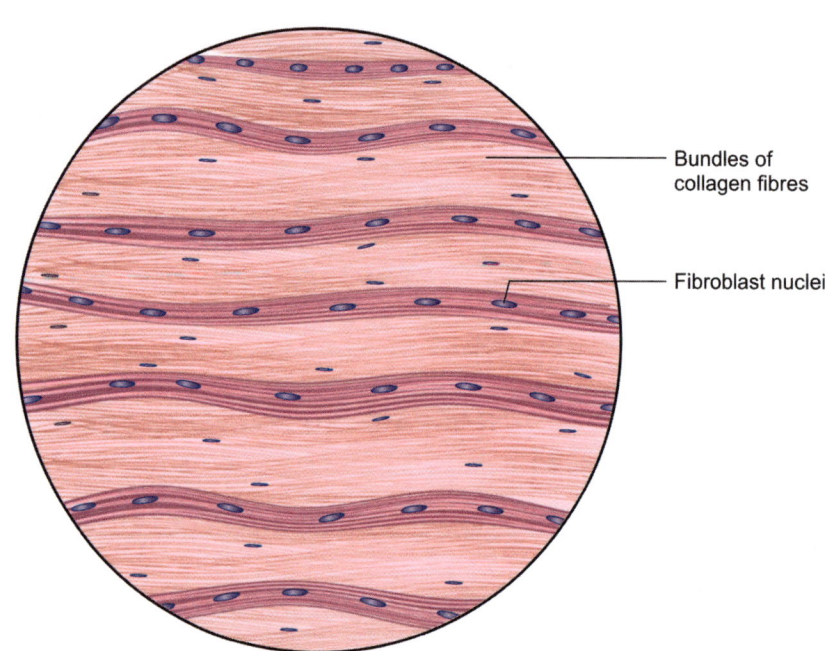

Tendon. Stain: Haematoxylin-eosin, 100X

Specialised regular dense connective tissue, e.g. cartilage and bone, described in Chapter 4.

Ordinary Irregular Dense Connective Tissue

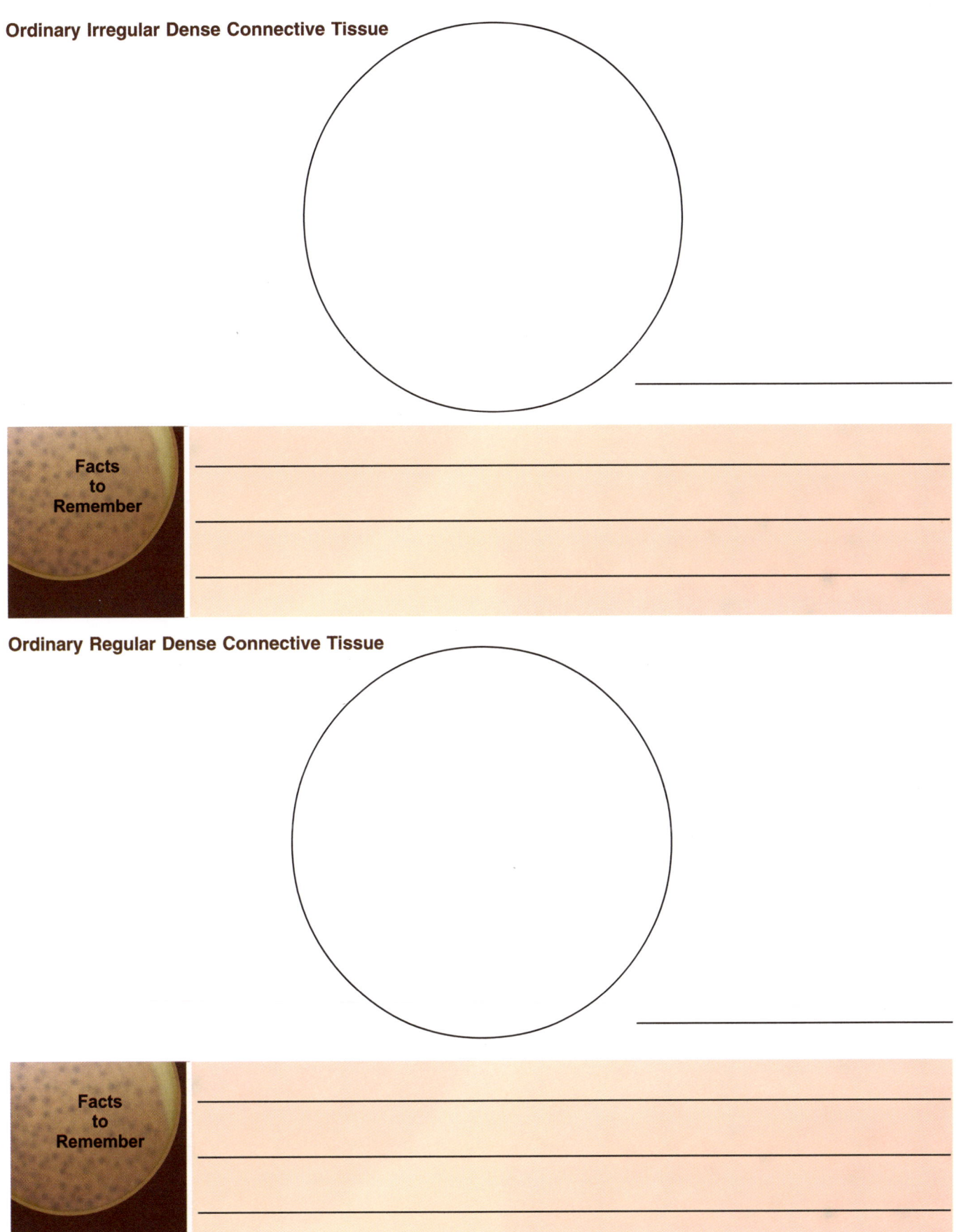

**Facts
to
Remember**

_____

_____

_____

Ordinary Regular Dense Connective Tissue

**Facts
to
Remember**

_____

_____

_____

4. Skeletal Tissue: Cartilage and Bone

Cartilage is a specialised dense connective tissue. It comprises cells, ground substance and fibres. Growth in cartilage occurs by:

a. Appositional growth: By surface deposition from the cells of inner perichondrial layer.

b. Interstitial growth: By the multiplication of cells situated within the matrix of the cartilage.

HYALINE CARTILAGE
Features

i. _____

ii. _____

iii. _____

_____

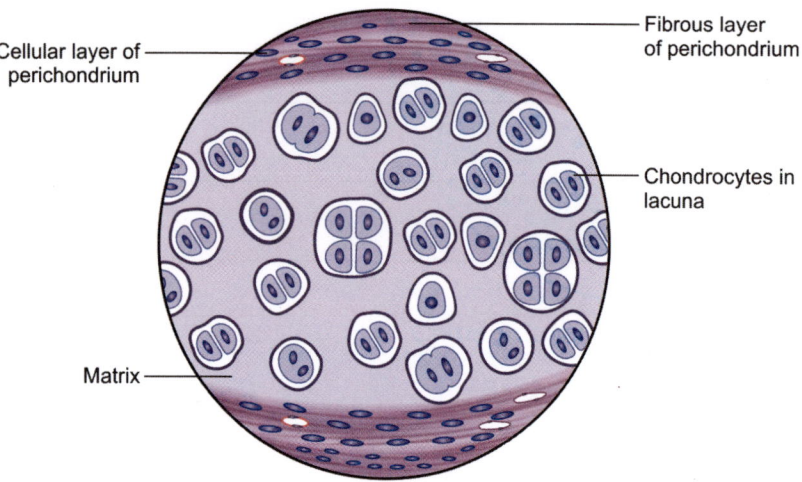

Trachea. Stain: Haematoxylin-eosin, 100X

Elastic Cartilage

i. _____

ii. _____

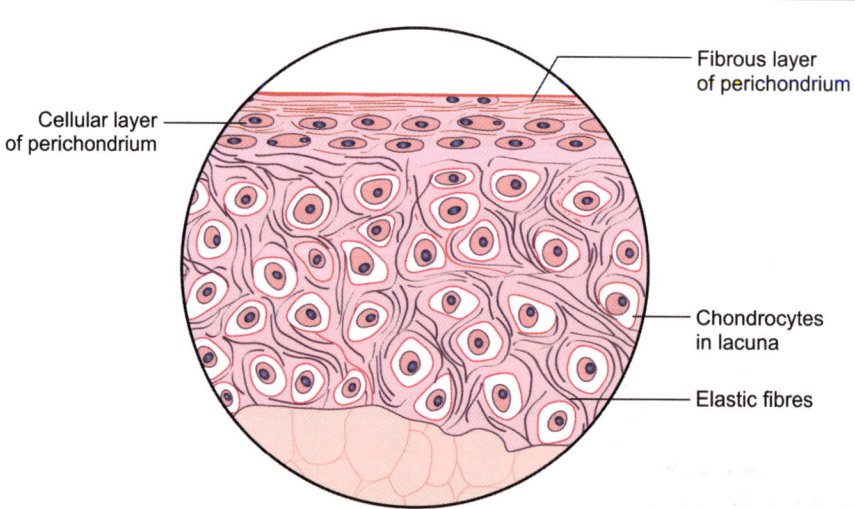

Epiglottis. Stain: Haematoxylin-eosin, 100X

Hyaline Cartilage

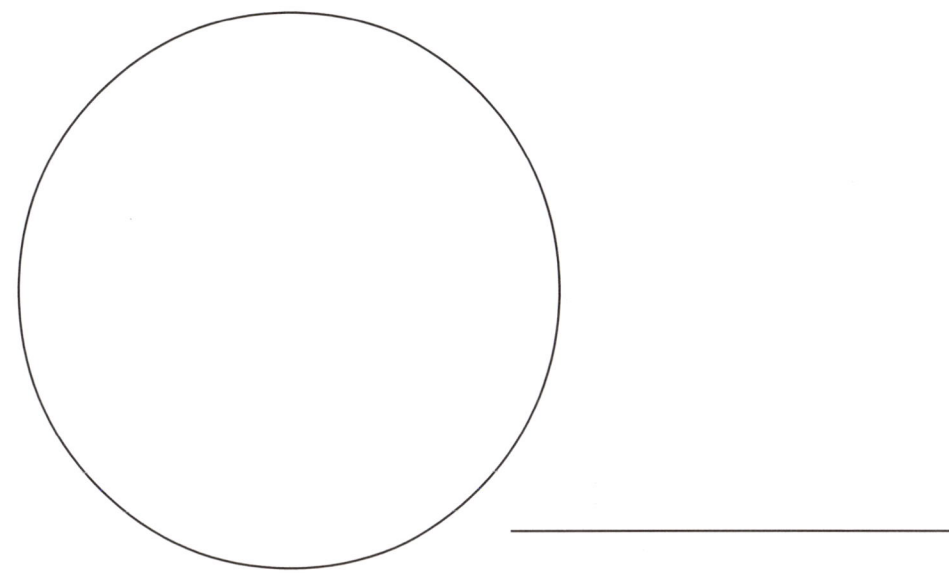

_____

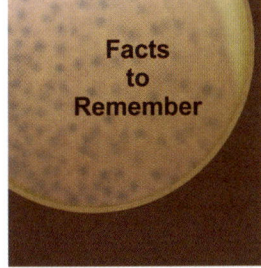

Facts to Remember

_____

_____

_____

Elastic Cartilage

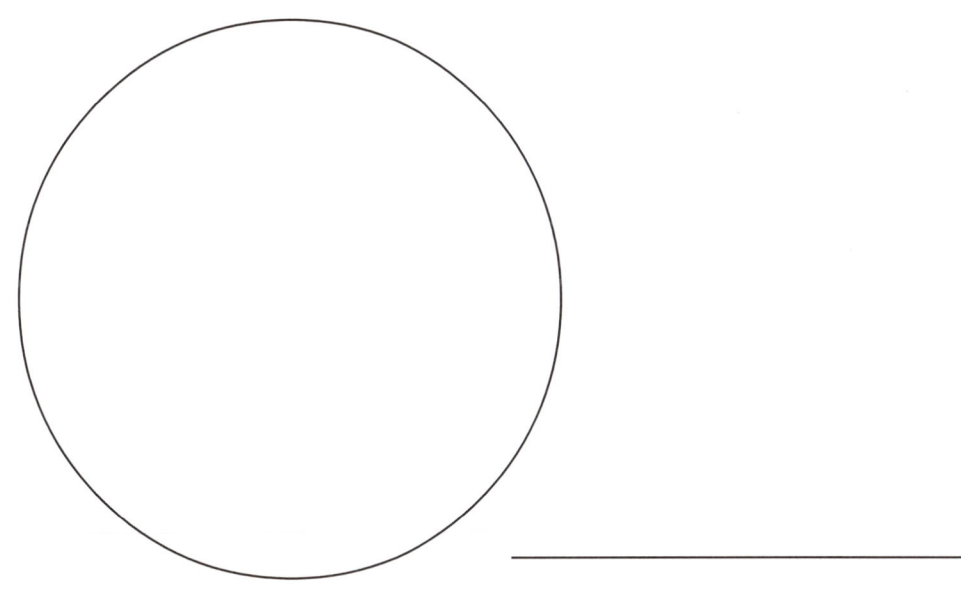

_____

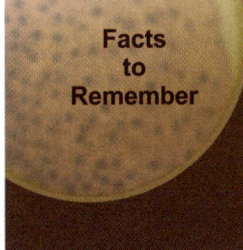

Facts to Remember

_____

_____

_____

FIBROCARTILAGE

Features

1. _____

_____

2. _____

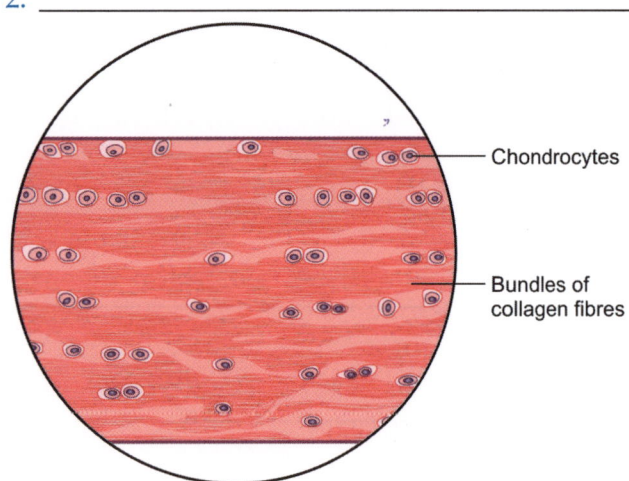

Intervertebral disc. Stain: Haematoxylin-eosin, 100X

BONE

Bone is another specialised dense connective tissue, where the matrix is impregnated with calcium salts making it hard and rigid. The calcium salts exist in the form of hydroxyapatite crystals [$Ca_{10}(PO_4)_6(OH)_2$] in the form of 'plates or rods'. Matrix is the complex of organic and inorganic intercellular substances which surrounds the osteocytes in a bone.

Compact Bone

Characteristic histologic feature of compact bone is haversian system or osteon.

a. _____

b. _____

c. _____

_____

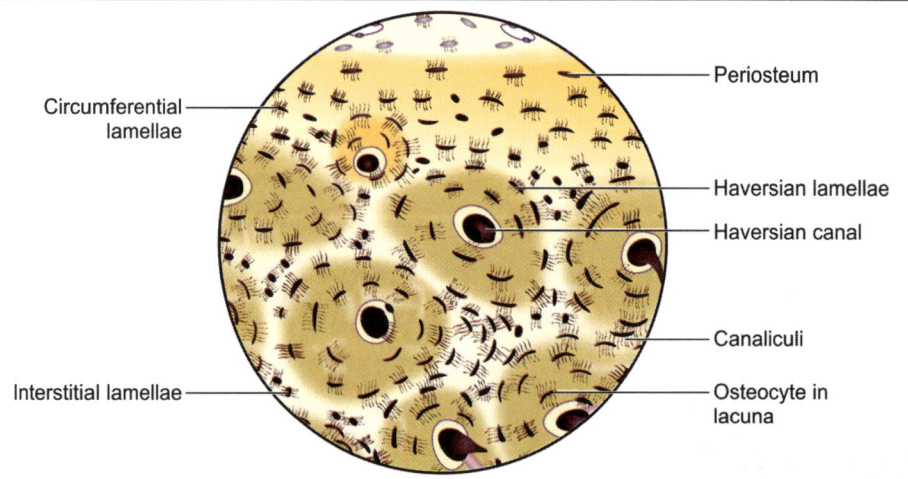

Shaft of a long bone. Stain: Haematoxylin-eosin, 100X

Fibrocartilage

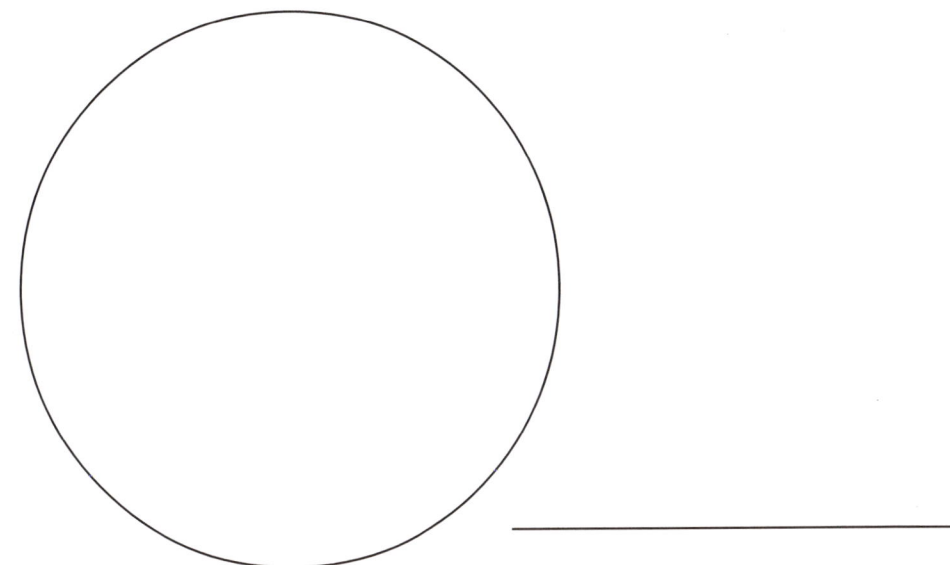

_____

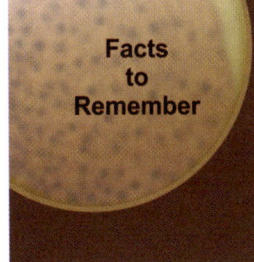

Facts to Remember

_____

_____

_____

Compact Bone

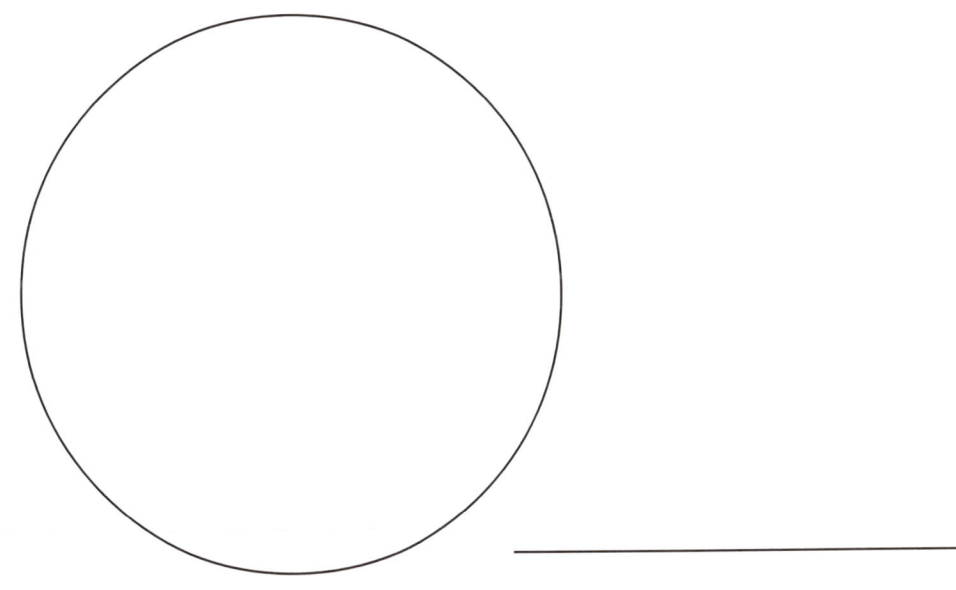

_____

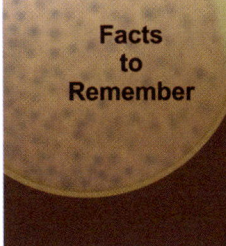

Facts to Remember

_____

_____

_____

Cancellous/Spongy Bone

Cancellous bone is covered with the periosteum. Haversian systems are absent in spongy bone. It consists of:

_____

_____

_____

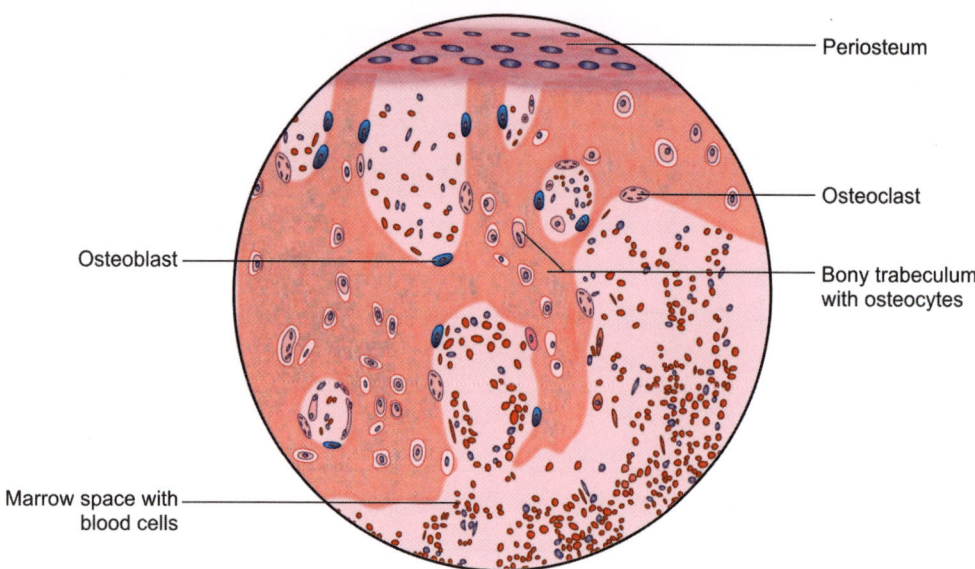

Sternum. Stain: Haematoxylin-eosin, 100X

Intracartilaginous Ossification

The long and short bones of the skeleton are ossified in cartilage. The first sign of ossification is that the cartilage cells or chondrocytes arrange themselves in columns shown in the figure below.

_____

_____

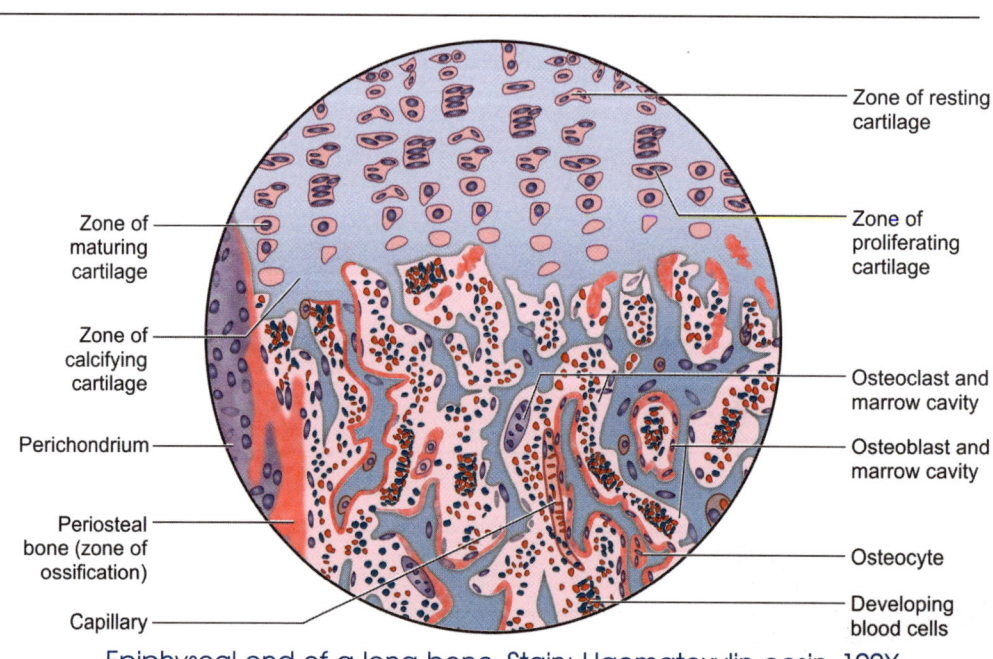

Epiphyseal end of a long bone. Stain: Haematoxylin-eosin, 100X

Cancellous/Spongy Bone

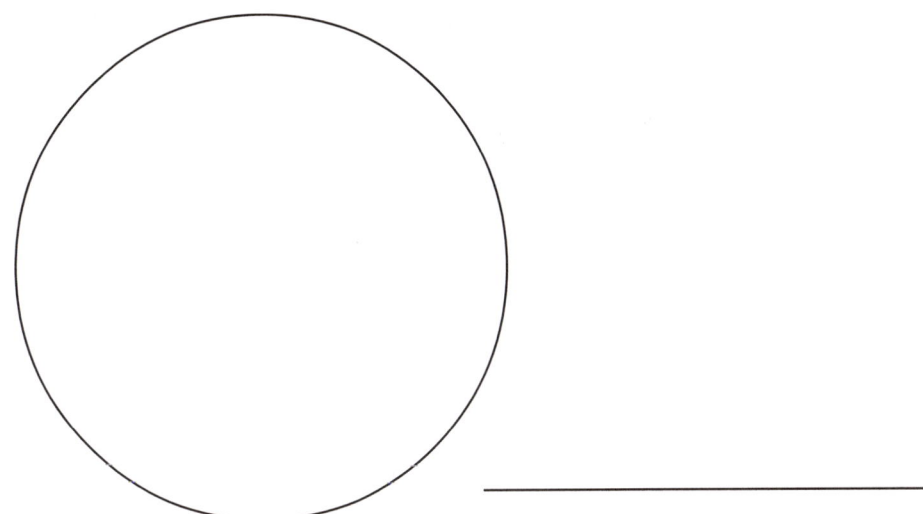

_____

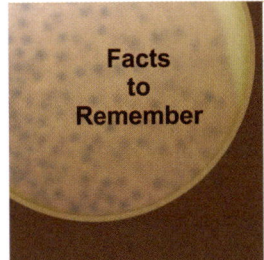

Facts to Remember

_____

_____

_____

Intracartilaginous Ossification

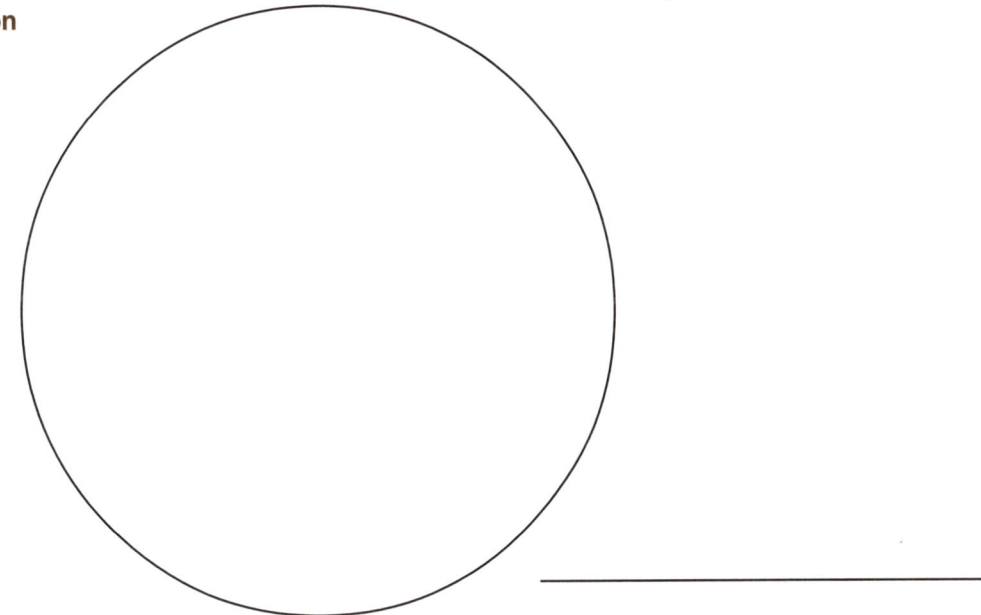

_____

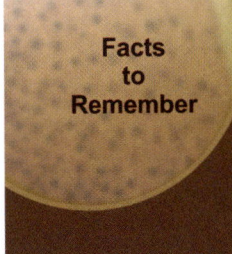

Facts to Remember

_____

_____

_____

ADDITIONAL FIGURES/NOTES

ADDITIONAL FIGURES/NOTES

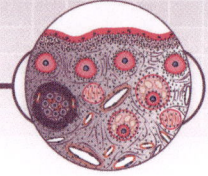

5. Muscular Tissue

Muscular tissue is responsible for movement of various parts of body with respect to one another. All muscles comprise elongated cells are called fibres.

Types

1. _____
2. _____
3. _____

Skeletal Muscle (Transverse section)

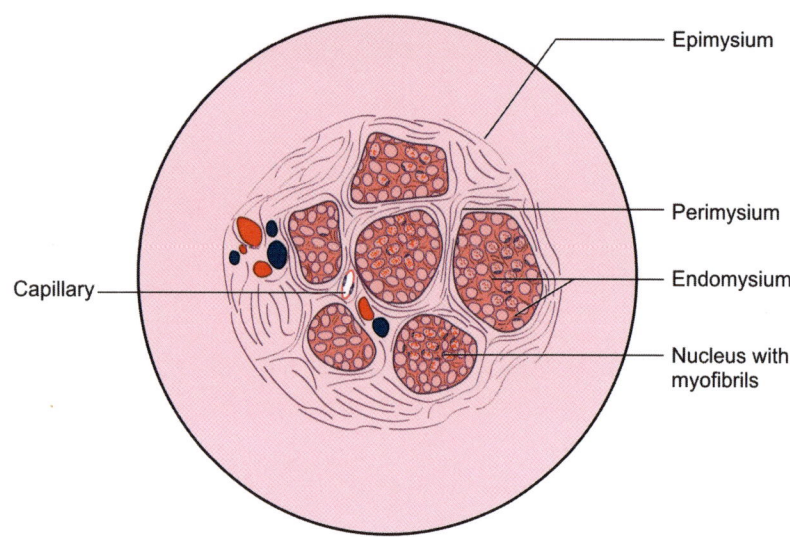

Deltoid muscle (transverse section). Stain: Haematoxylin-eosin, 100X

Striated/Skeletal Muscle (Longitudinal section)

_____

_____

_____

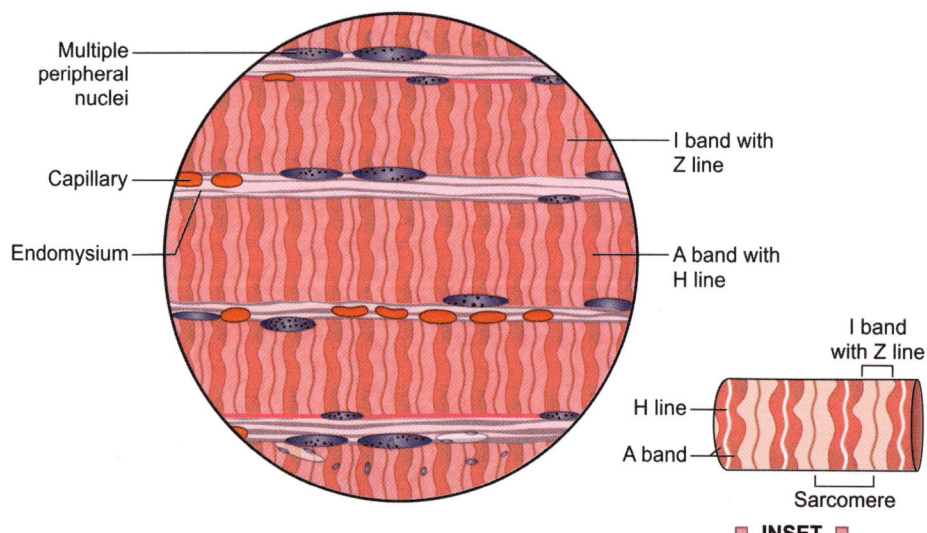

Deltoid muscle (longitudinal section). Stain: Haematoxylin-eosin, 400X

Skeletal Muscle (Transverse section)

Facts to Remember

Striated/Skeletal Muscle (Longitudinal section)

Facts to Remember

Smooth Muscle

_____

_____

_____

_____

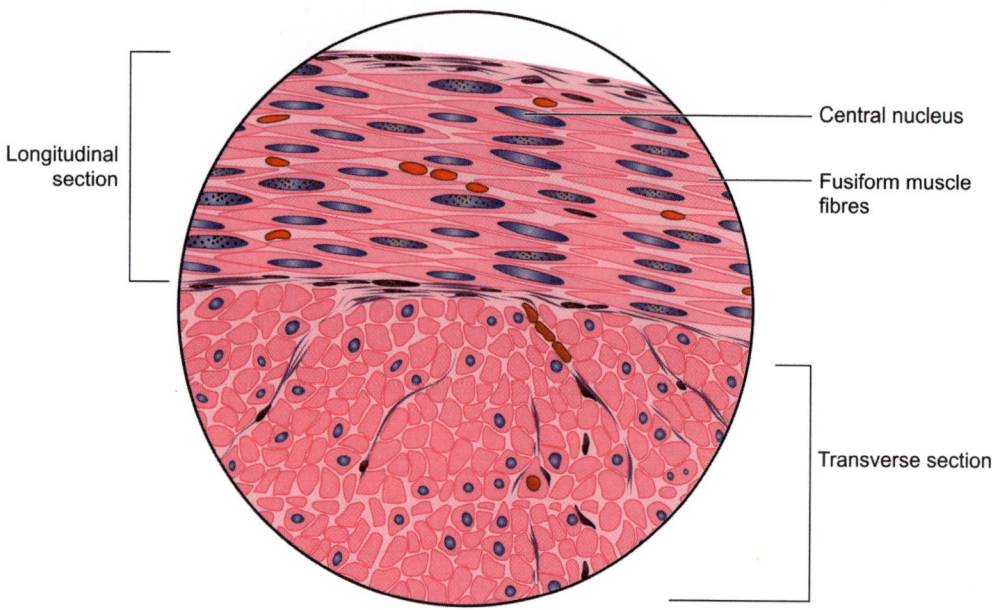

Longitudinal section

Central nucleus

Fusiform muscle fibres

Transverse section

Stomach. Stain: Haematoxylin-eosin, 100X

Cardiac Muscle

_____

_____

_____

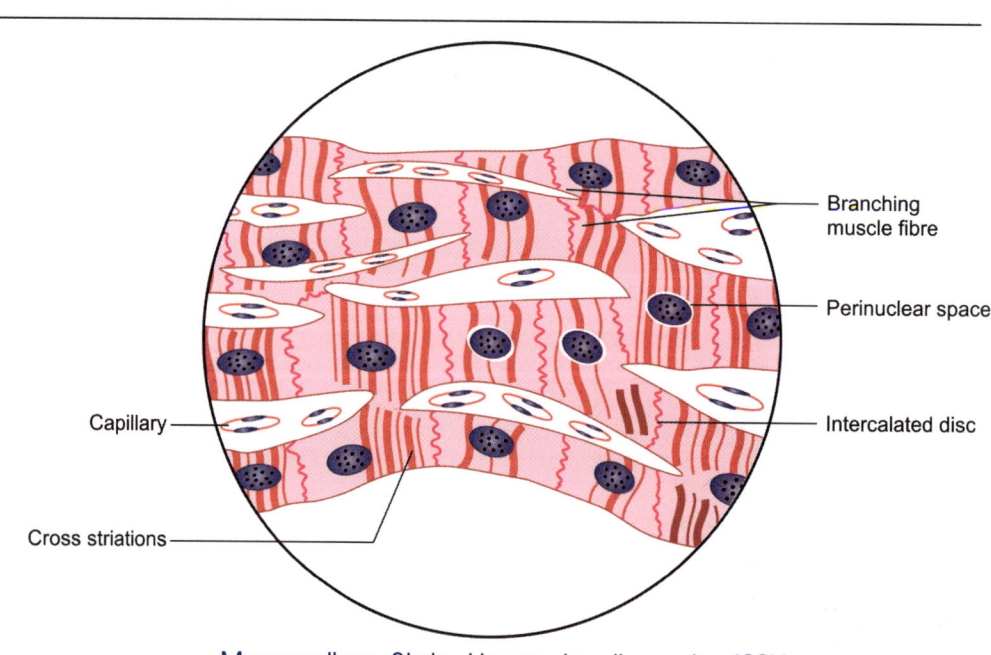

Branching muscle fibre

Perinuclear space

Intercalated disc

Capillary

Cross striations

Myocardium. Stain: Haematoxylin-eosin, 400X

Smooth Muscle

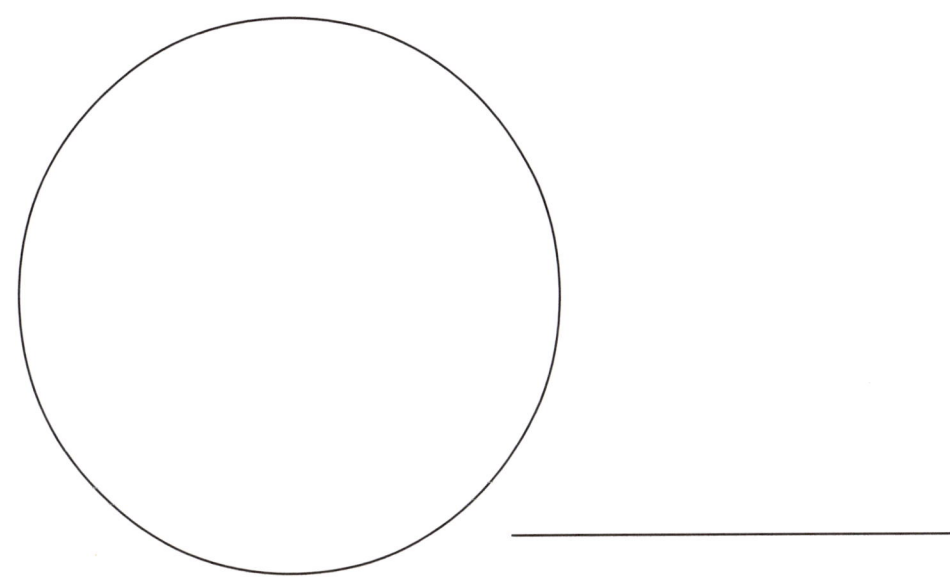

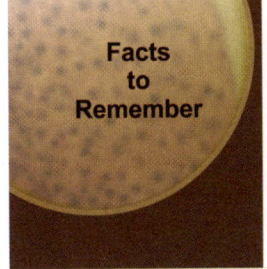

Facts
to
Remember

Cardiac Muscle

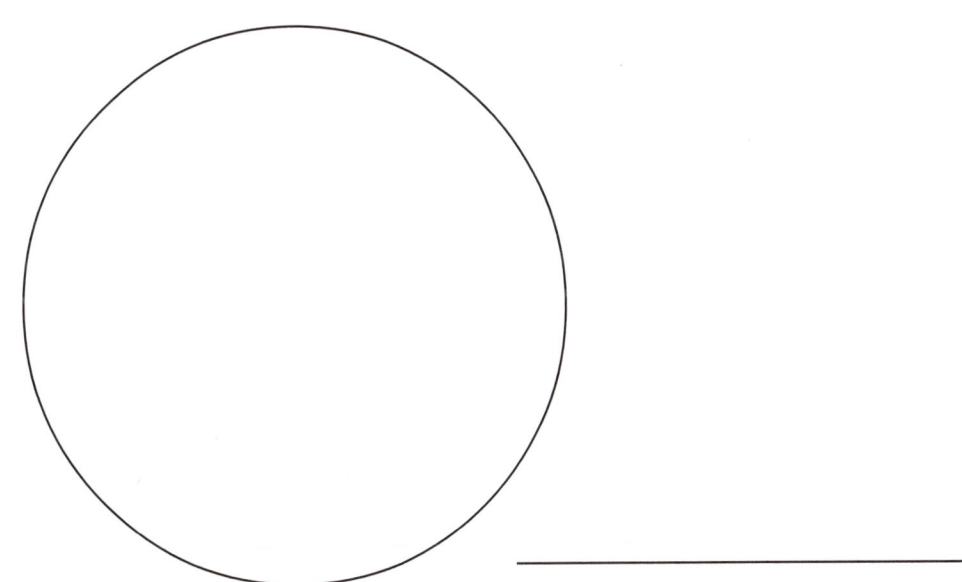

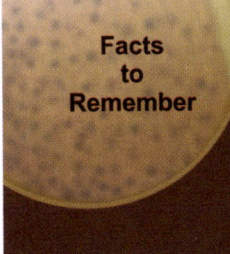

Facts
to
Remember

6. Nervous Tissue

Nervous tissue is the specialised tissue responsible for excitability and conduction of impulses. Nervous tissue comprises: Neuron, i.e. nerve cells with its processes; and neuroglia the cellular connective tissue of the nervous system.

NEURON

Neuron is the structural and functional unit of nervous tissue.

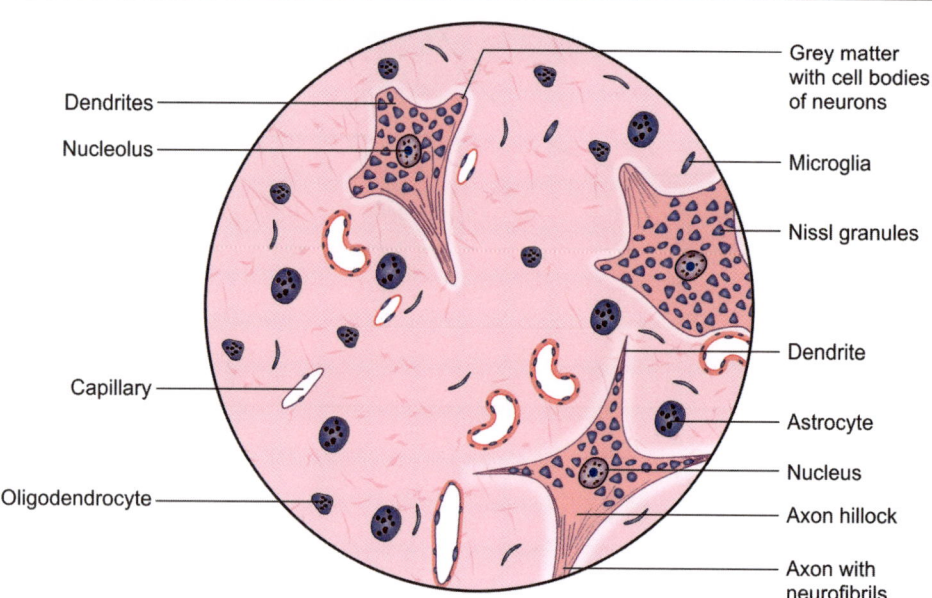

Grey matter of spinal cord. Stain: Haematoxylin-eosin, 400X

SPINAL CORD

The spinal cord comprises a central canal surrounded by grey matter. Around this grey matter is the white matter.

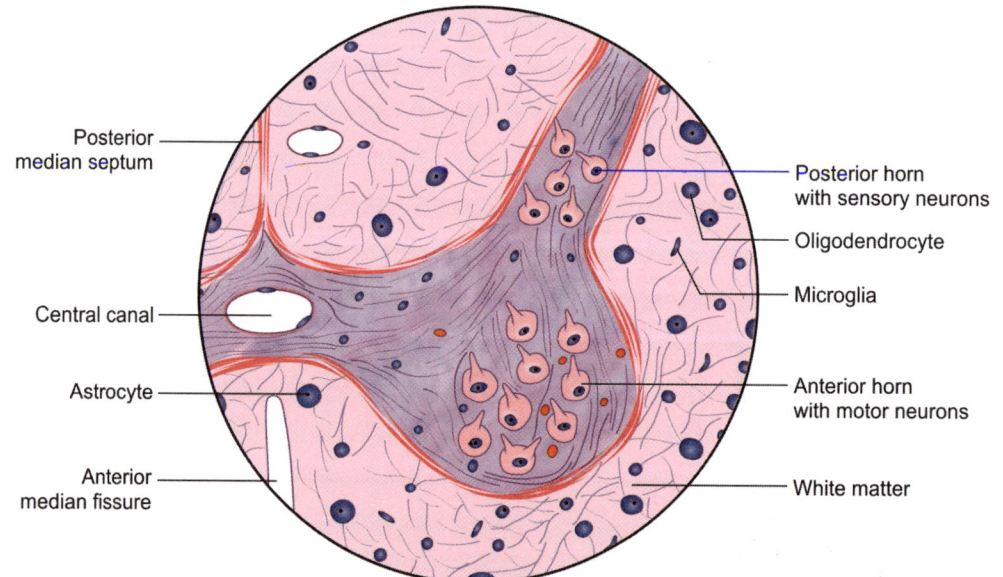

Spinal cord. Stain: Haematoxylin-eosin, 100X

Neuron

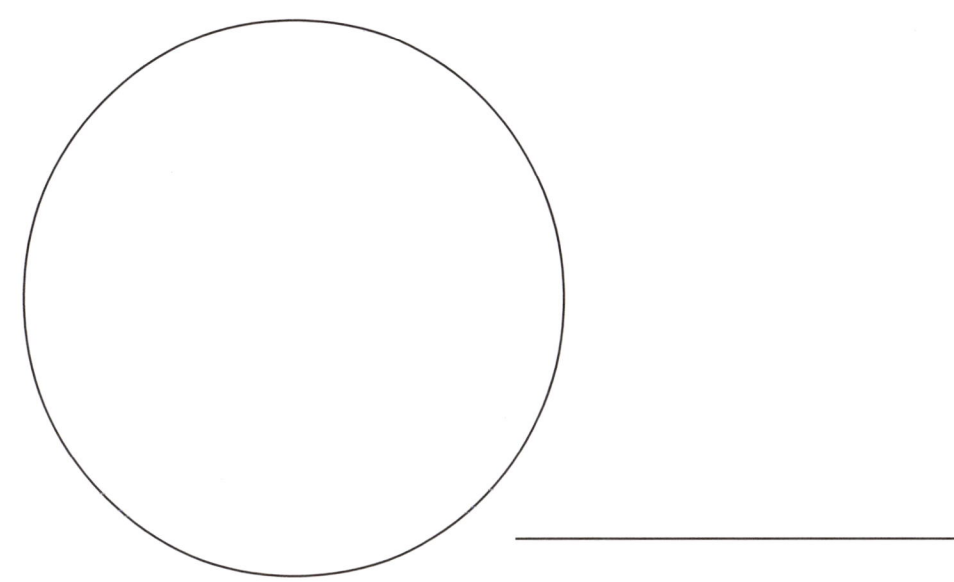

_____

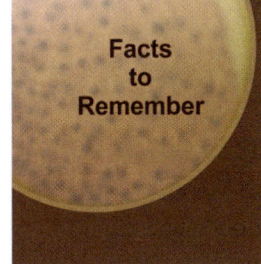

Facts to Remember

_____

_____

_____

Spinal Cord

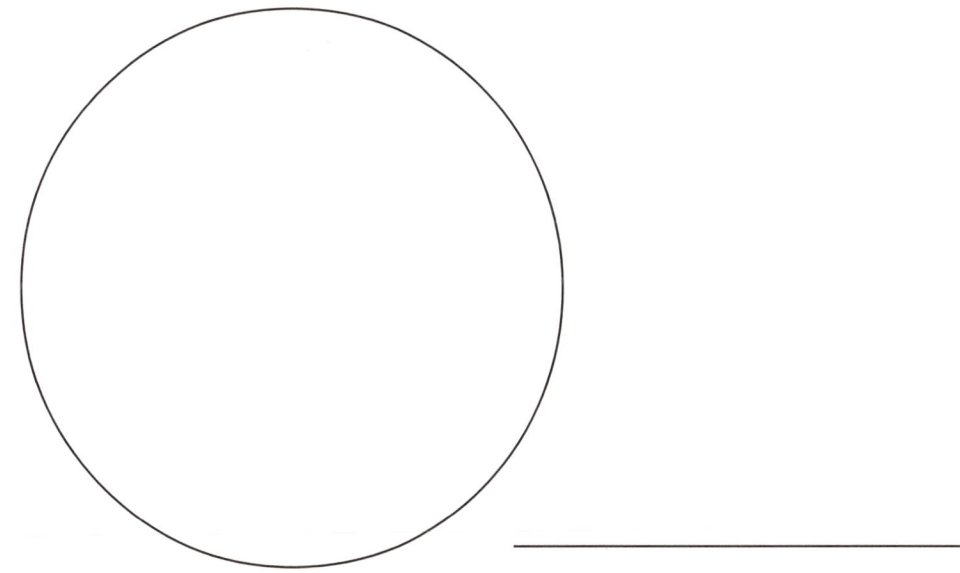

_____

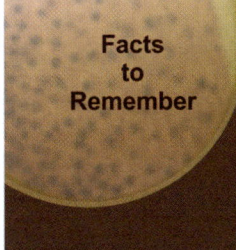

Facts to Remember

_____

_____

_____

White Matter of Spinal Cord, Ganglia and Nerves

The white matter of spinal cord consists of nerve fibres and neuroglia. Various cells of neuroglia are:

Astrocytes: _____

Oligodendrocytes: _____

Microglia: _____

Ependymal cells: _____

Satellite or capsular cells: _____

Schwann's cells: _____

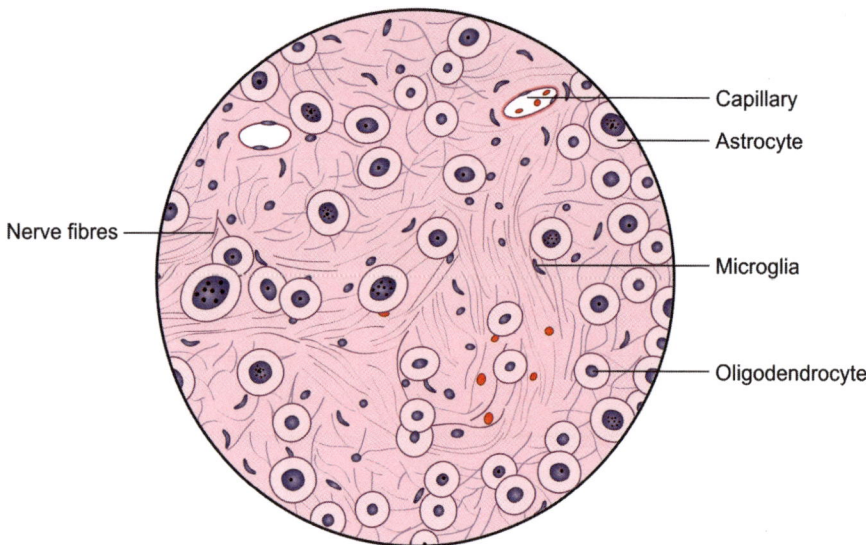

White matter of spinal cord. Stain: Haematoxylin-eosin, 100X

NERVE FIBRE

A peripheral nerve fibre is an axon/dendron with its covering, i.e. myelin sheath stained by osmic acid and neurilemma. These fibres are myelinated. Each fibre consists of: _____

_____

_____

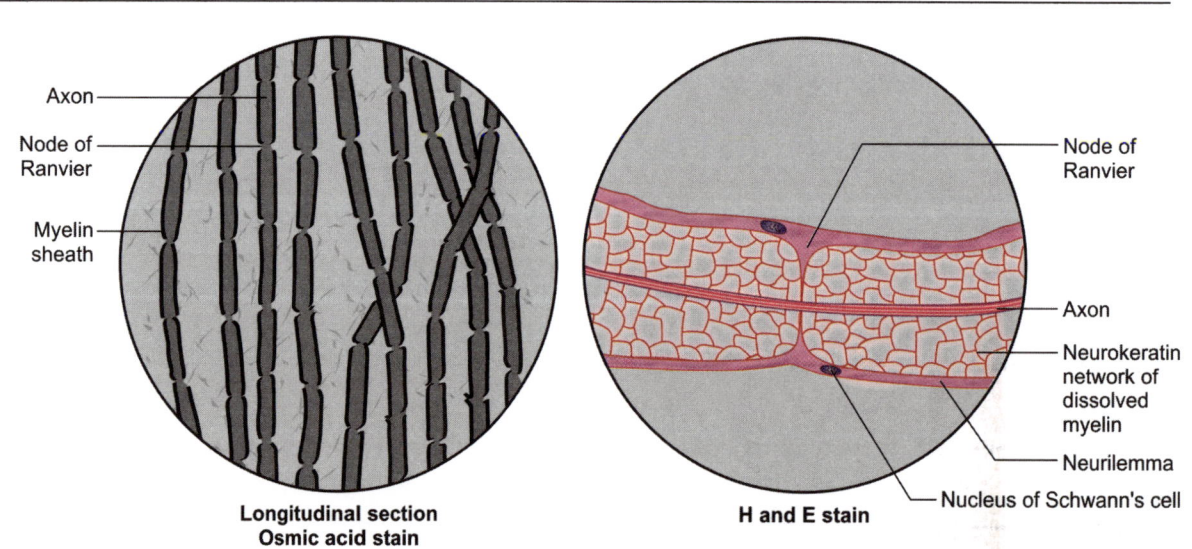

Longitudinal section
Osmic acid stain

H and E stain

Myelinated nerve fibre, 100X

White Matter of Spinal Cord

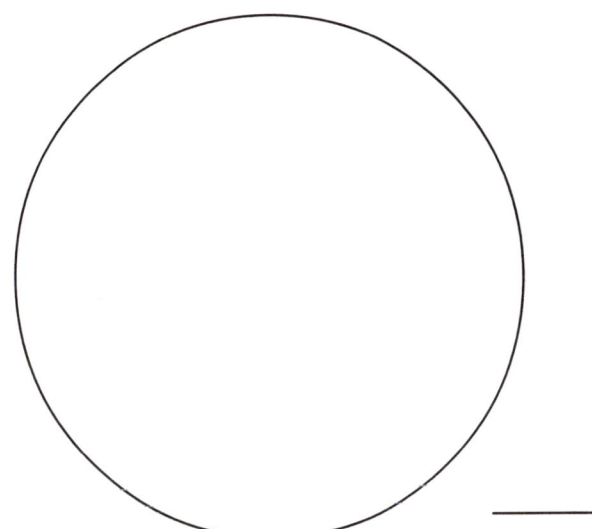

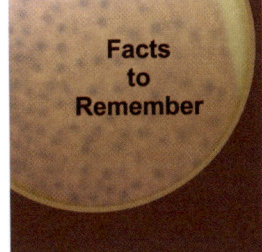

**Facts
to
Remember**

_____

_____

_____

_____

Nerve Fibre: Longitudinal Section

Osmic acid stain

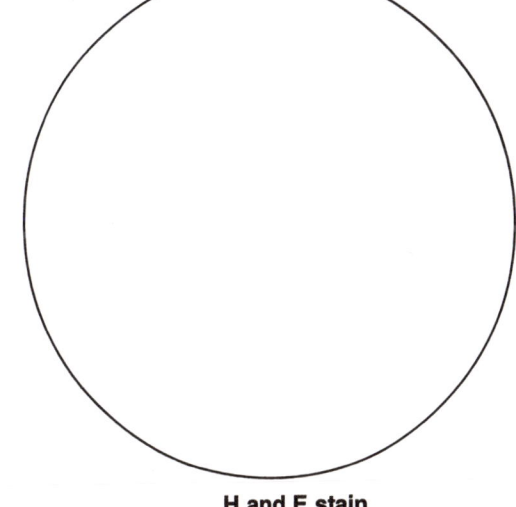

H and E stain

**Facts
to
Remember**

_____

_____

_____

Transverse section of nerve trunk: The nerve trunk is surrounded by epineurium; each fasciculus is surrounded by perineurium and around each fibre is endoneurium. Osmic acid only stains the myelin sheath.

_____

_____

_____

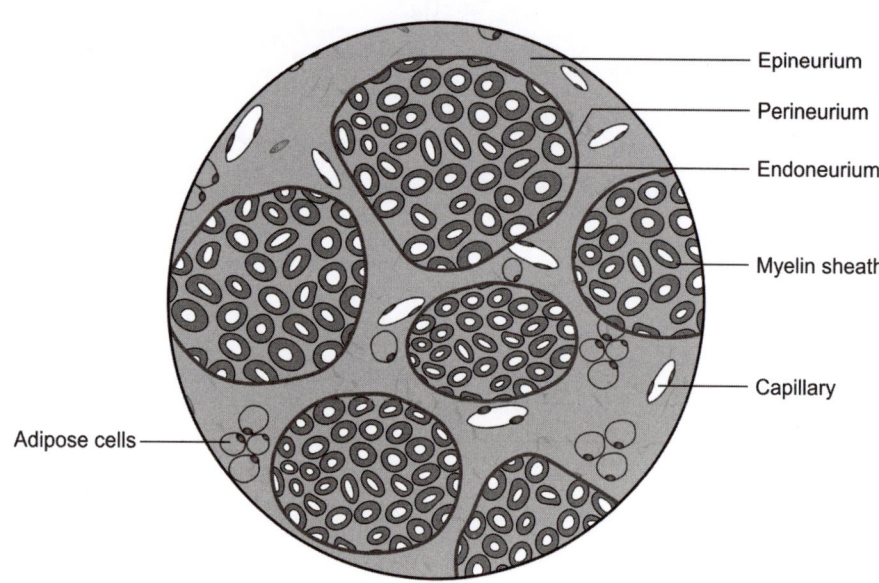

Nerve trunk. Stain: Osmic acid, 100X

H and E stains the axon and the neurilemma. Myelin sheath is not stained by H and E stain.

_____

_____

_____

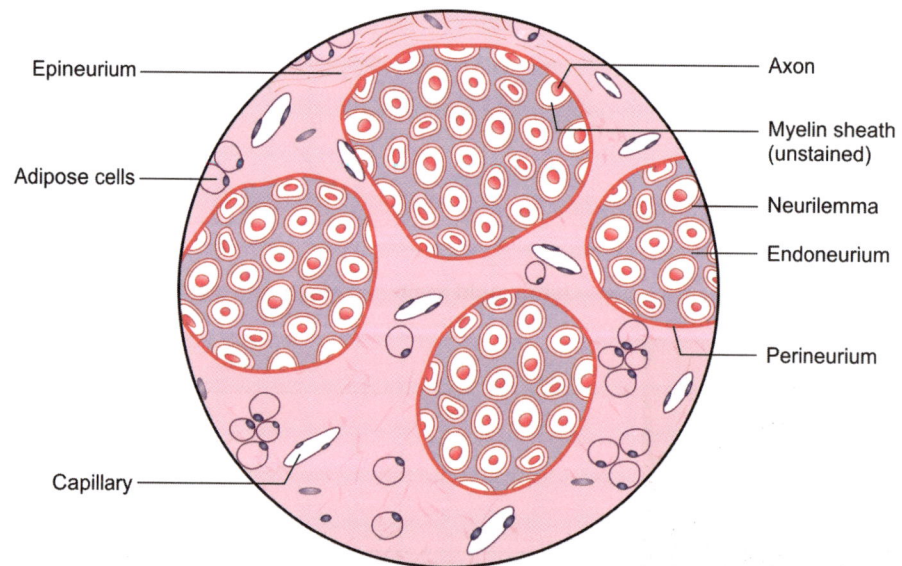

Nerve trunk. Stain: Haematoxylin-eosin, 100X

**Transverse Section of Nerve Trunk
(Osmic acid stain)**

**Facts
to
Remember**

**Transverse Section of Nerve Trunk
(H and E stain)**

**Facts
to
Remember**

GANGLIA

Collection of neurons outside the central nervous system is called ganglion. There are two types of ganglia, spinal and autonomic.

Spinal/Sensory/Dorsal Root Ganglion

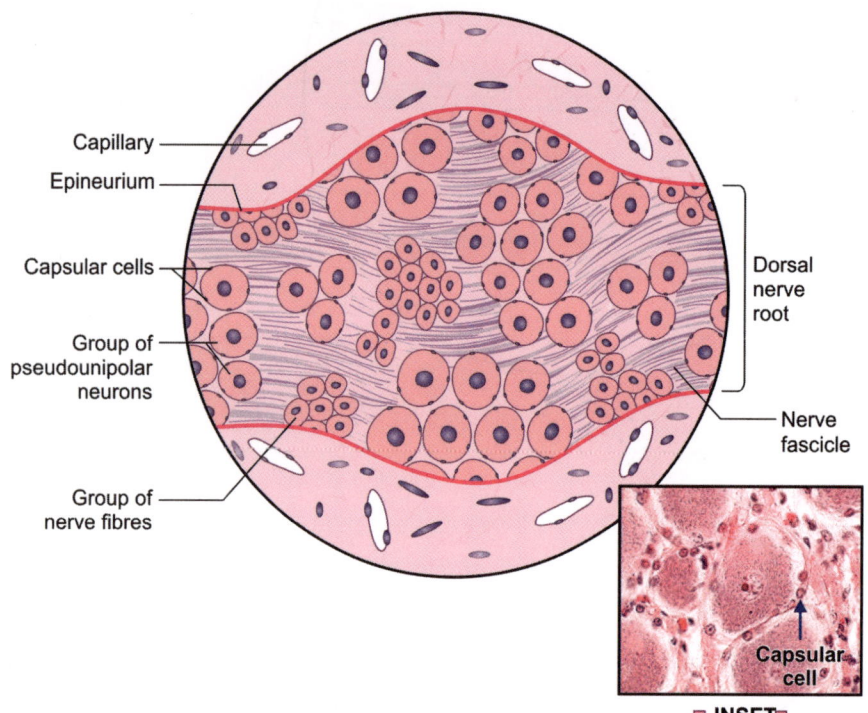

Spinal ganglion. Stain: Haematoxylin-eosin, 400X

Autonomic Ganglion

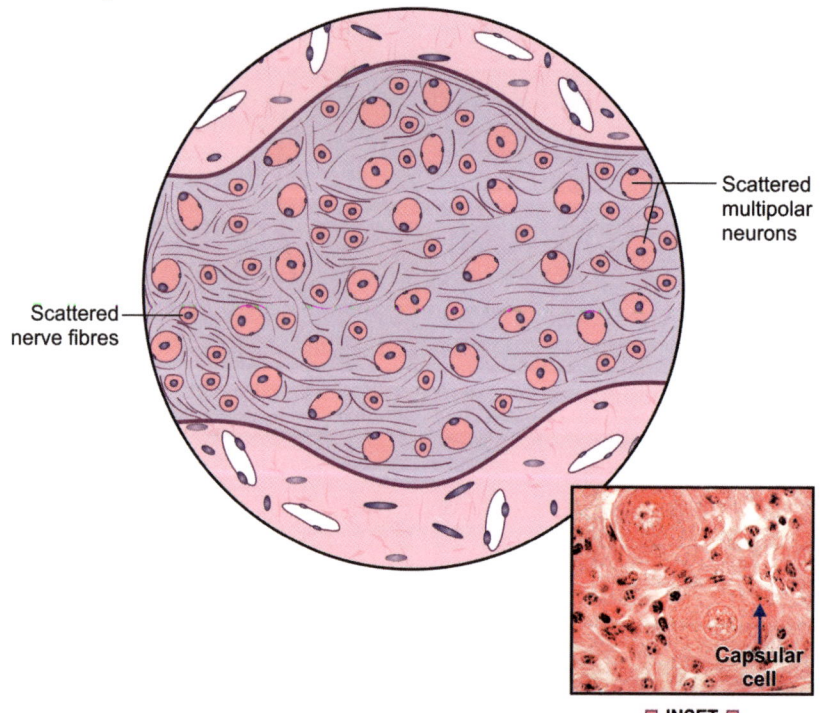

Autonomic ganglion. Stain: Haematoxylin-eosin, 400X

Spinal/Sensory/Dorsal Root Ganglion

**Facts
to
Remember**

Autonomic Ganglion

**Facts
to
Remember**

CEREBRUM

It is characterised by *heterotypical cortex*, i.e. histological structure differs in various regions of cerebral cortex. From superficial to deep, the following six layers are shown in the figure. These layers are:

_____

_____

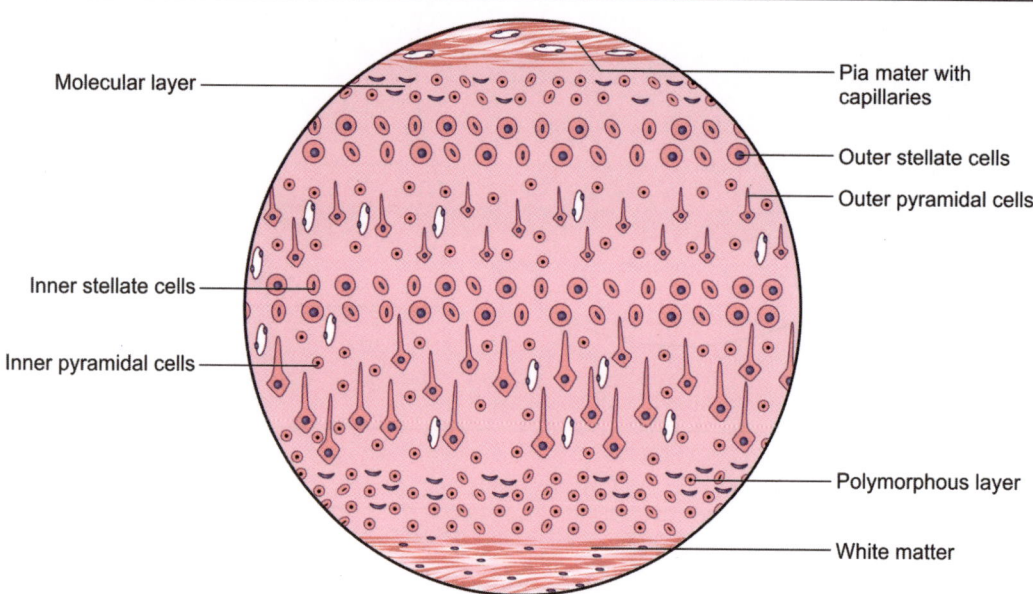

Molecular layer

Inner stellate cells

Inner pyramidal cells

Pia mater with capillaries

Outer stellate cells

Outer pyramidal cells

Polymorphous layer

White matter

Grey matter. Stain: Haematoxylin-eosin, 400X

CEREBELLUM

The histological structure of entire cerebellum is similar and is called *homotypical cortex*. The cerebellar cortex shows many deep folds called *cerebellar folia*, separated by fissures. The cerebellum consists of outer grey matter and inner white matter. The layers of grey matter are:

_____

_____

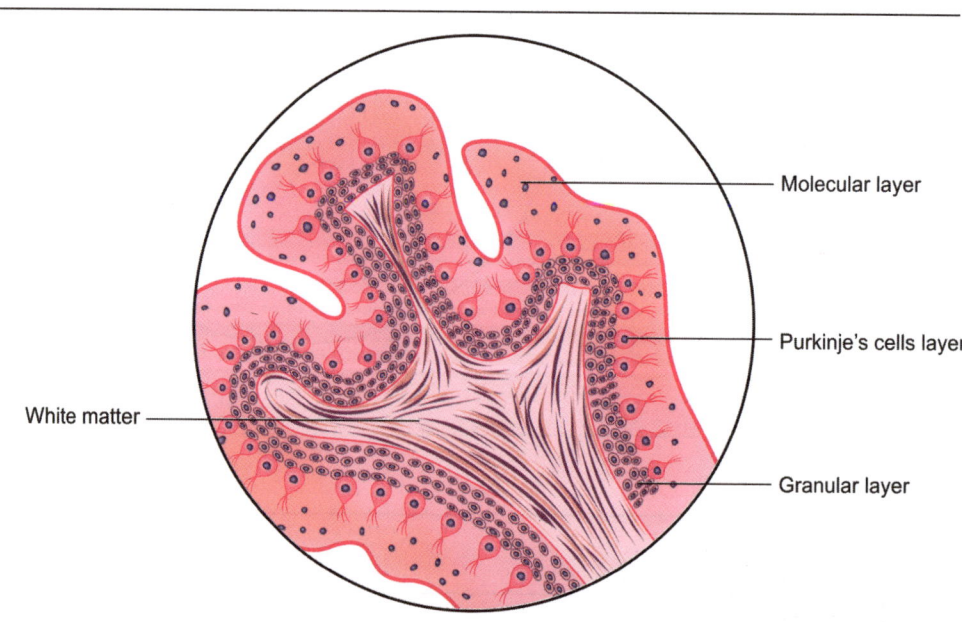

Molecular layer

Purkinje's cells layer

White matter

Granular layer

Cerebellar cortex. Stain: Haematoxylin-eosin, 100X

Cerebrum

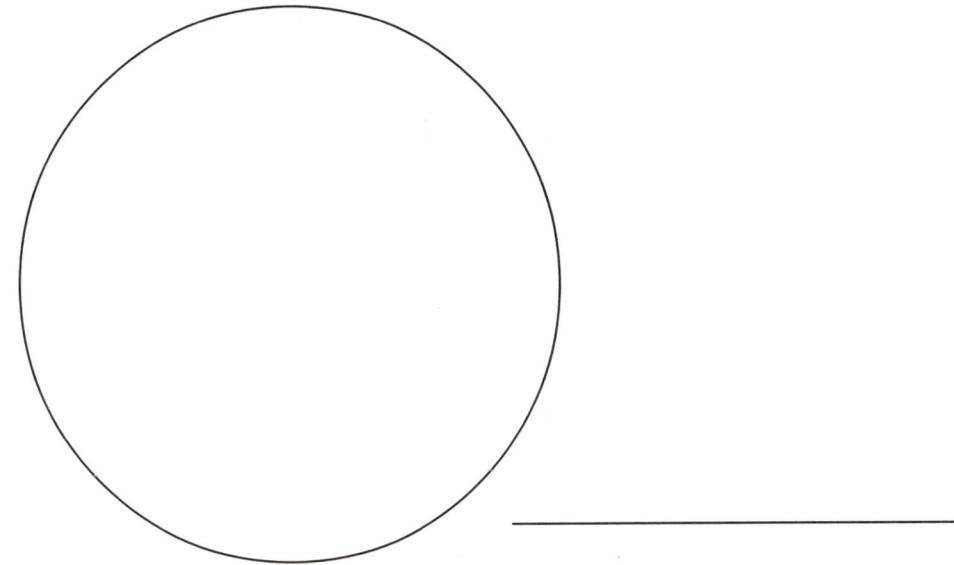

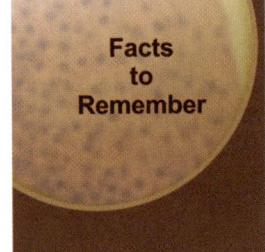

Facts to Remember

Cerebellum

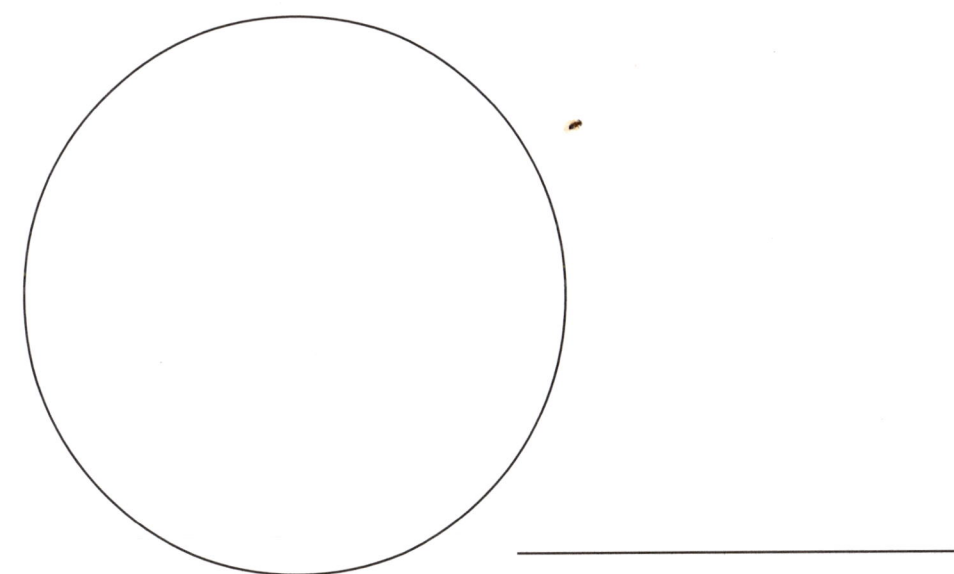

Facts to Remember

ADDITIONAL FIGURES/NOTES

ADDITIONAL FIGURES/NOTES

7. Blood Vessels

Main blood vessels are: (1) arteries and (2) veins.

ARTERIES

Arteries are classified as: Elastic, muscular and arterioles.

a. *Elastic arteries:* _____

_____

_____

_____

_____

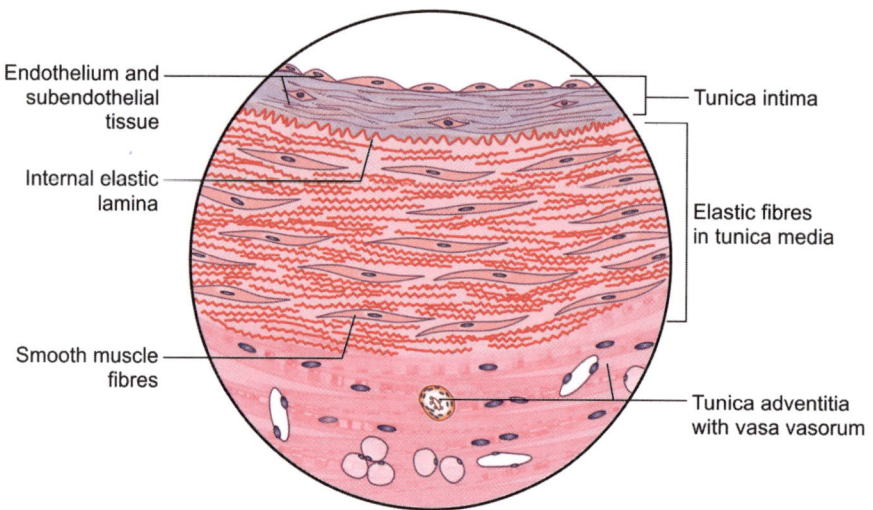

Endothelium and
subendothelial
tissue

Internal elastic
lamina

Smooth muscle
fibres

Tunica intima

Elastic fibres
in tunica media

Tunica adventitia
with vasa vasorum

Aorta. Stain: Haematoxylin-eosin, 100X

b. *Muscular arteries:* _____

_____

_____

_____

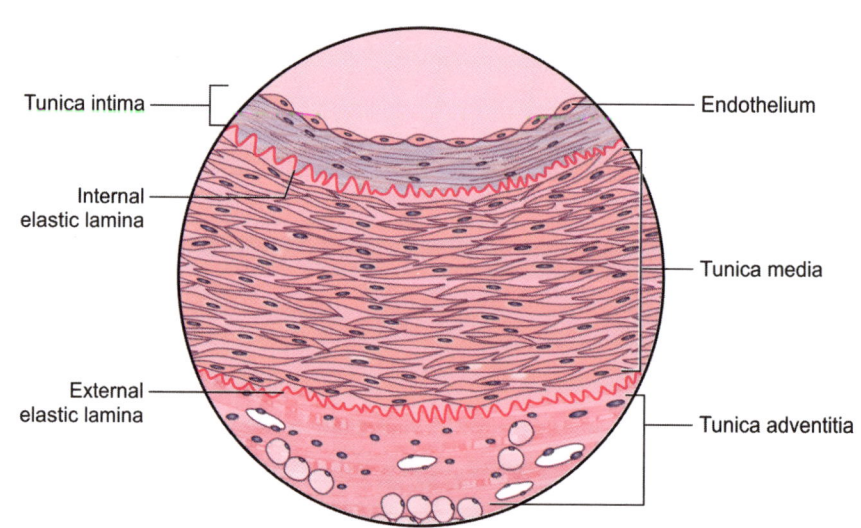

Tunica intima

Internal
elastic lamina

External
elastic lamina

Endothelium

Tunica media

Tunica adventitia

Brachial artery. Stain: Haematoxylin-eosin, 100X

Elastic Arteries

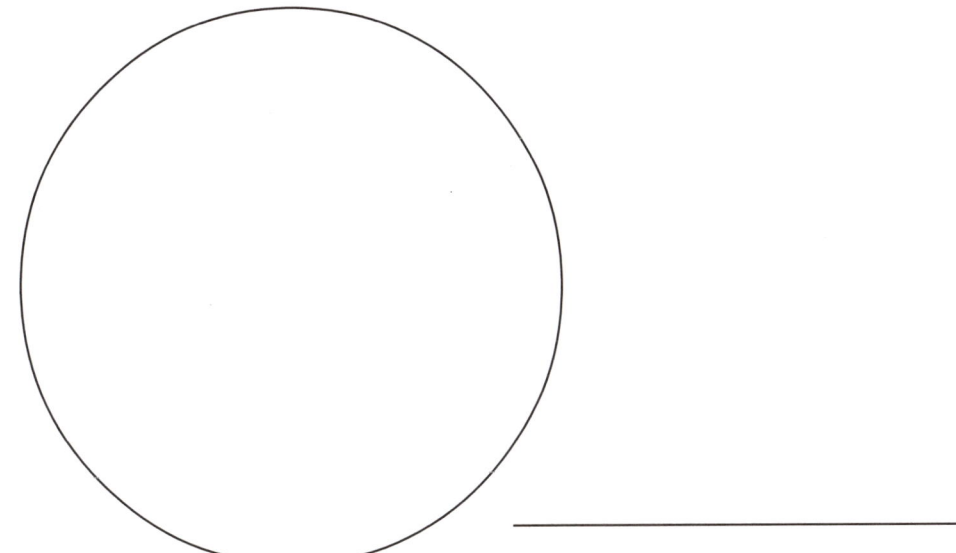

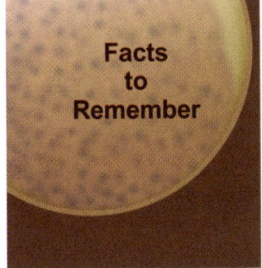

Facts to Remember

Muscular Arteries

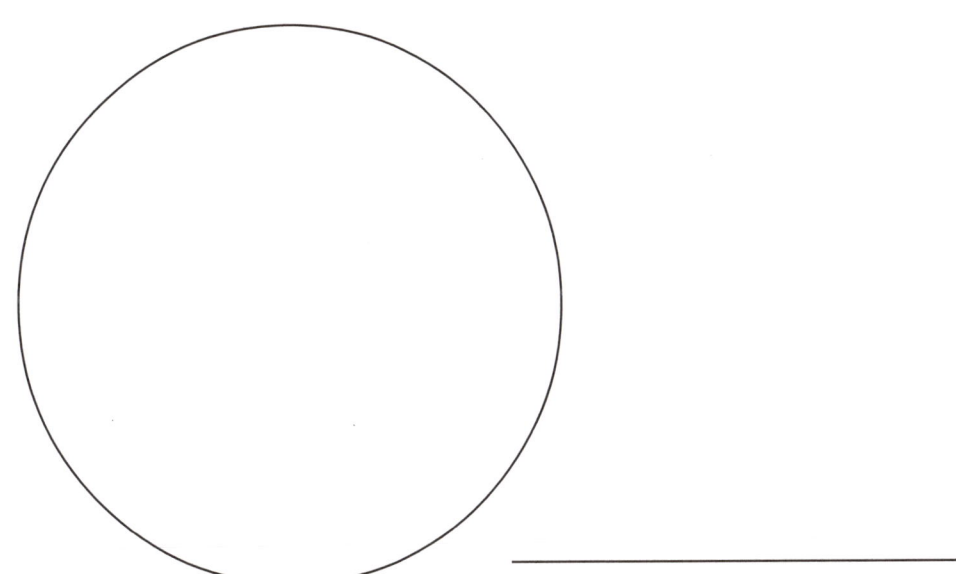

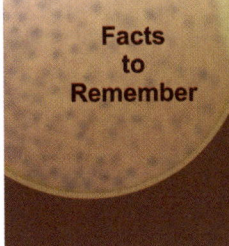

Facts to Remember

c. *Arterioles:* These are the smallest divisions of the arteries which have a diameter of **100 micron**. These act as resistance vessels to maintain peripheral blood pressure. Three concentric coats surrounding the lumen are (i) tunica intima, (ii) tunica media, and (iii) tunica adventitia.

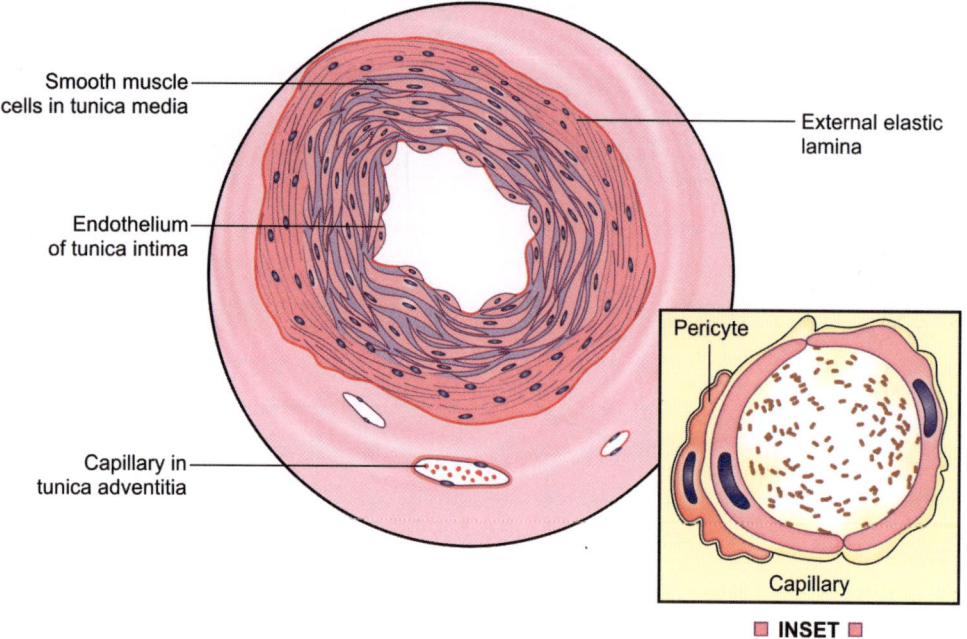

Smooth muscle cells in tunica media

External elastic lamina

Endothelium of tunica intima

Pericyte

Capillary in tunica adventitia

Capillary

☐ **INSET** ☐

Arteriole and capillary. Stain: Haematoxylin-eosin, 100X

VEINS

These are vessels which collect and bring deoxygenated blood to the heart, exceptions being the umbilical, and pulmonary veins. Its layers are: _____

_____

_____

_____

_____

_____

Endothelium

Tunica media (1/3rd)

Blood in lumen

Tunica adventitia (2/3rd)

Basilic vein. Stain: Haematoxylin-eosin, 100X

Arterioles

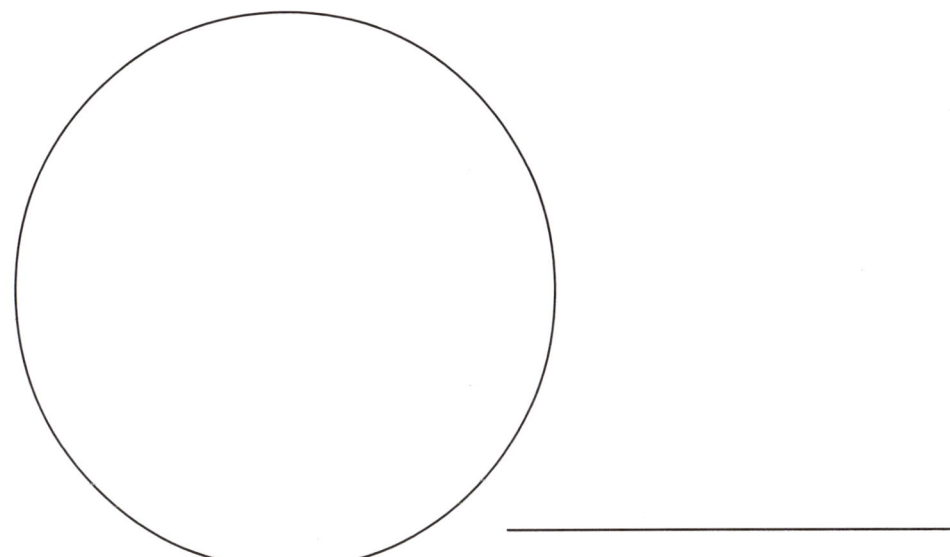

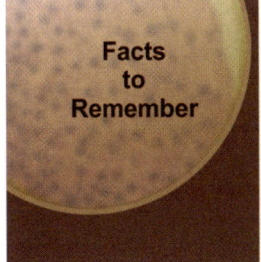

Facts to Remember

Veins

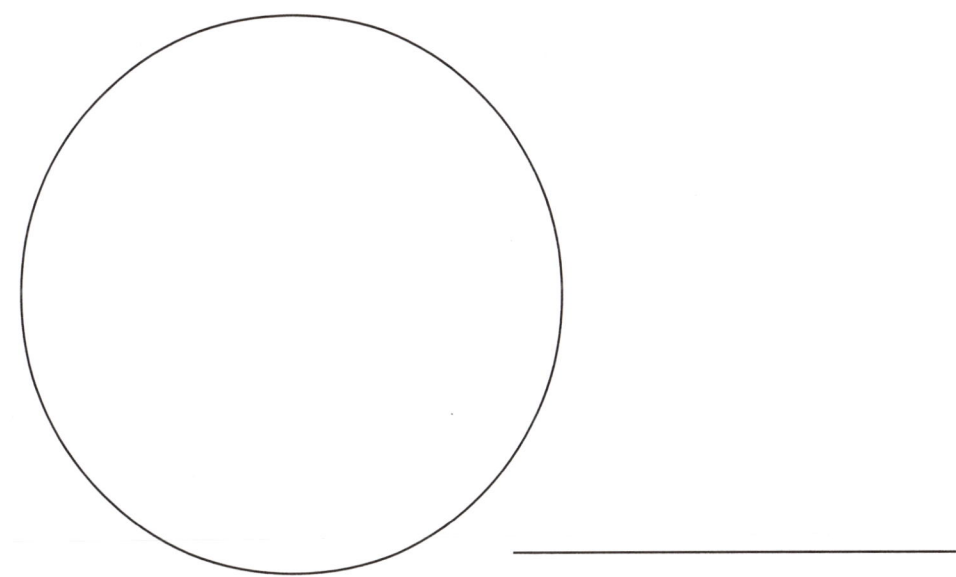

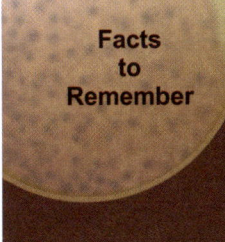

Facts to Remember

8. Lymphatic Organs

Lymph node, spleen, thymus and tonsil.

STRUCTURE OF LYMPH NODE

The cut surface of a lymph node is seen to be divided into an outer peripheral cortex and an inner medulla.

Cortex contains lymphatic nodules/primary nodules which are about 1 mm in diameter.

Medulla consists of lymphocytes arranged in cords called *medullary cords* which contain plasma cells, macrophages and small lymphocytes.

The thymus derived "T lymphocytes" are confined in the deep cortical (**paracortical**) region.

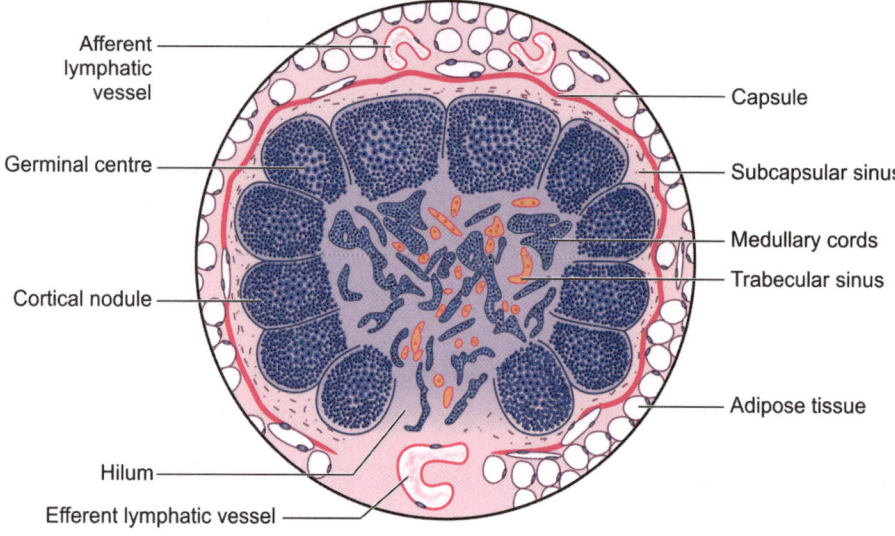

Afferent lymphatic vessel
Germinal centre
Cortical nodule
Hilum
Efferent lymphatic vessel
Capsule
Subcapsular sinus
Medullary cords
Trabecular sinus
Adipose tissue

Axillary lymph node. Stain: Haematoxylin-eosin, 100X

Magnified View of Lymph Nodules

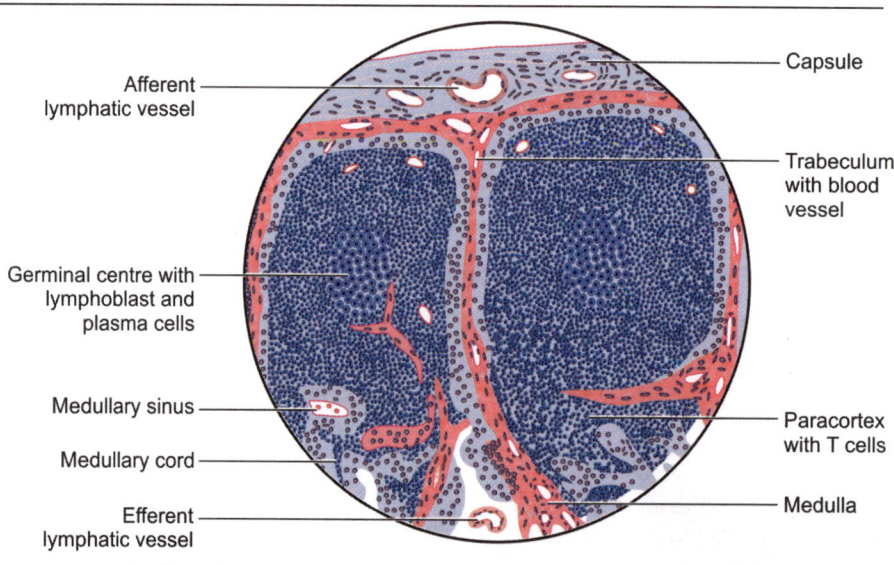

Afferent lymphatic vessel
Germinal centre with lymphoblast and plasma cells
Medullary sinus
Medullary cord
Efferent lymphatic vessel
Capsule
Trabeculum with blood vessel
Paracortex with T cells
Medulla

Axillary lymph node. Stain: Haematoxylin-eosin, 400X

Lymph Node

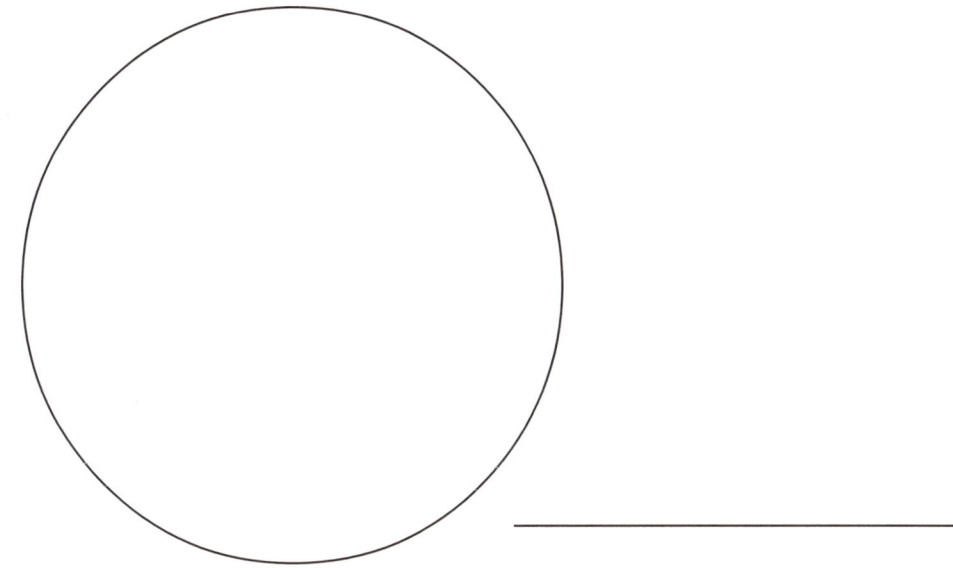

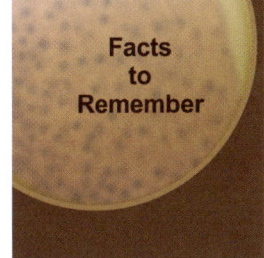

**Facts
to
Remember**

_____

_____

_____

Lymph Nodules

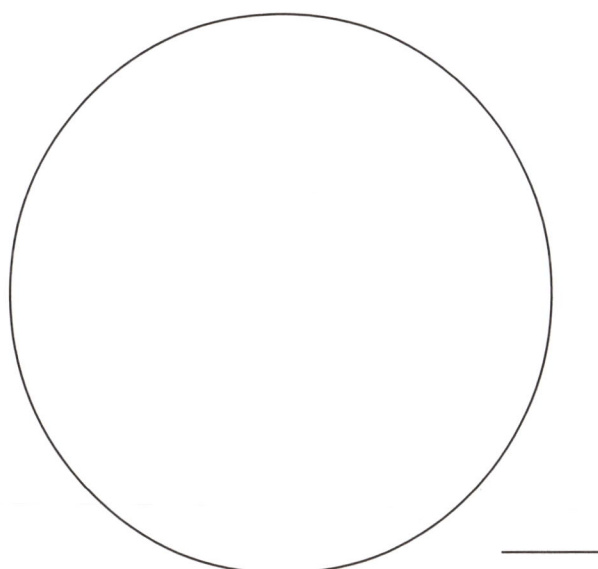

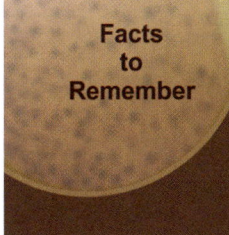

**Facts
to
Remember**

_____

_____

_____

SPLEEN

Spleen contains large amount of lymphatic tissue which **filters blood** instead of lymph. The spleen is comprised of **white pulp and red pulp**. White pulp is seen in the form of lymphatic nodules usually with an eccentric arteriole. The red pulp comprises a loose framework of reticular fibres with many lymphocytes, free macrophages, RBC, neutrophils and monocytes. "T zone of lymphocytes" is around the perivascular sheath.

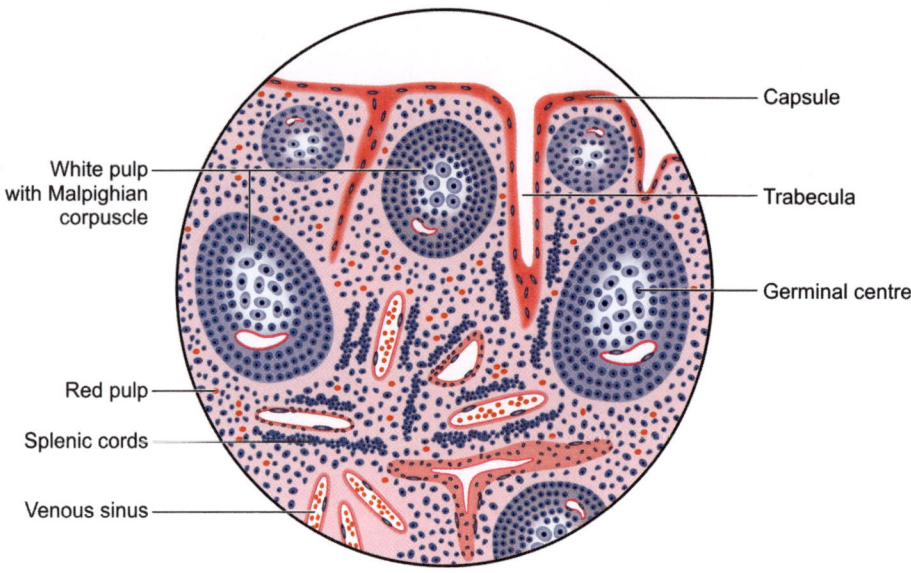

White pulp with Malpighian corpuscle

Red pulp

Splenic cords

Venous sinus

Capsule

Trabecula

Germinal centre

Spleen. Stain: Haematoxylin-eosin, 100X

Splenic Circulation

_____

_____

_____

_____

_____

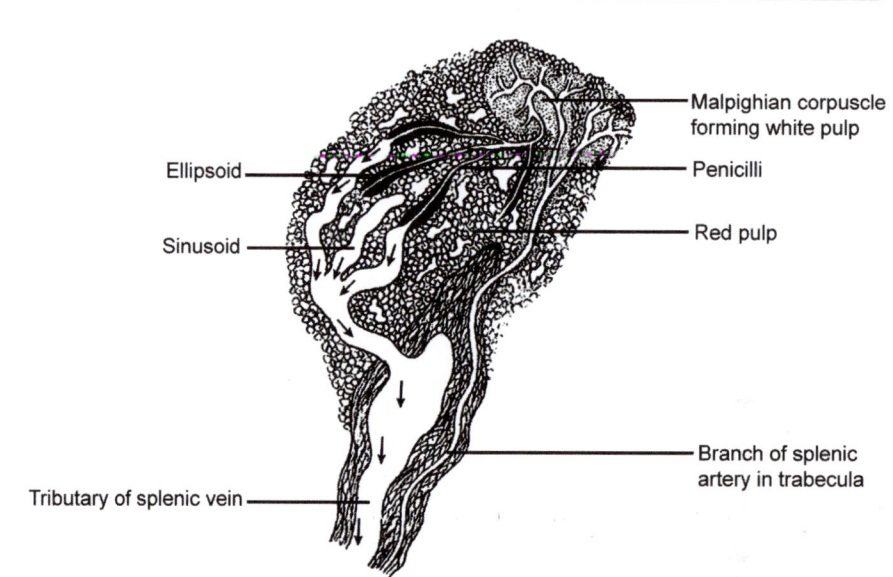

Ellipsoid

Sinusoid

Tributary of splenic vein

Malpighian corpuscle forming white pulp

Penicilli

Red pulp

Branch of splenic artery in trabecula

Splenic circulation

Spleen

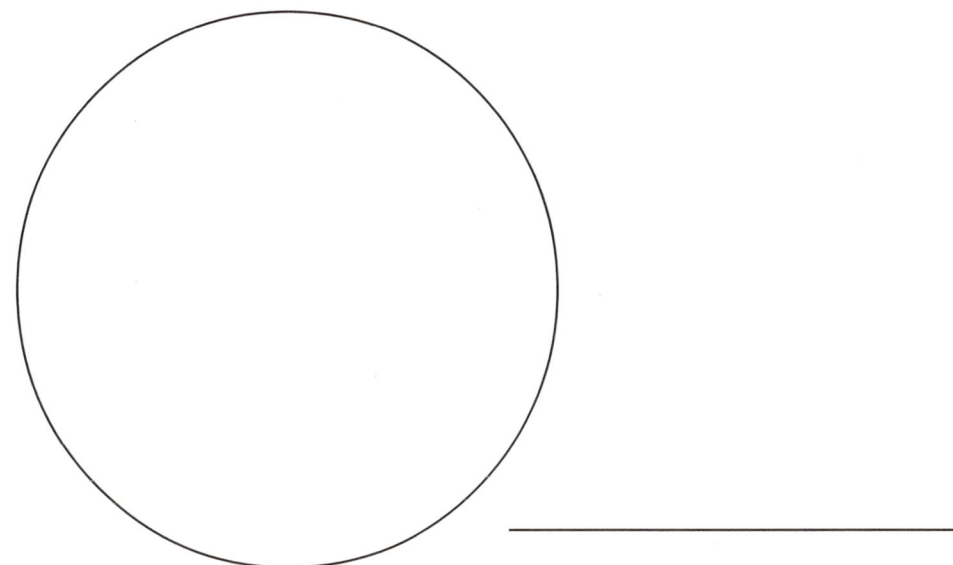

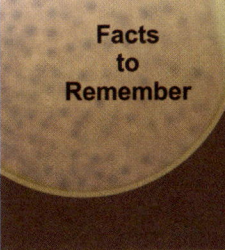
Facts
to
Remember

Splenic Circulation

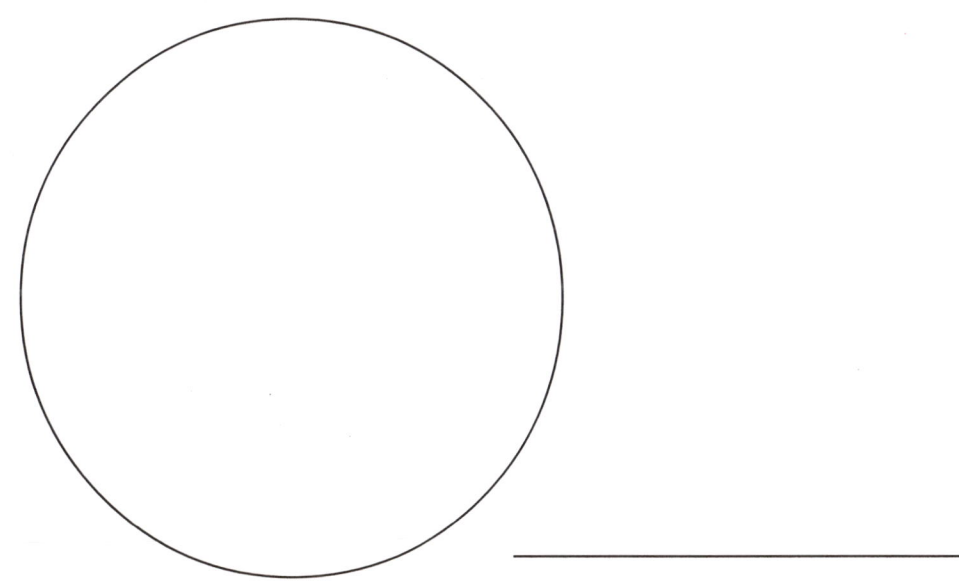

Facts
to
Remember

THYMUS

Thymus is a lymphoepithelial lobulated organ that produces "T lymphocytes" and a lymphocyte stimulating hormone. Thymus involutes at puberty. Each lobule has a peripheral darker cortex and a central lighter medulla. Since the septa do not extend into the medulla there is continuity of the medullary tissue of the various lobules. Chief cells are: *Thymic lymphocytes, epithelial reticular cells*. Hassall's corpuscles are formed by: _____

_____

_____

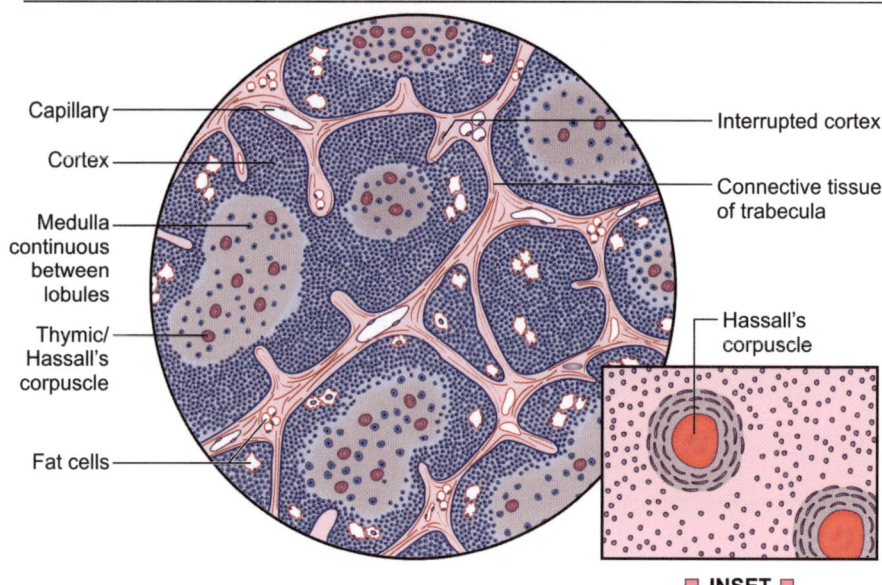

Capillary

Cortex

Medulla continuous between lobules

Thymic/ Hassall's corpuscle

Fat cells

Interrupted cortex

Connective tissue of trabecula

Hassall's corpuscle

■ INSET ■

Thymus at puberty. Stain: Haematoxylin-eosin, 100X

PALATINE TONSIL

It is a collection of paired lymphoid tissue at the oropharyngeal isthmus. Its oral aspect is covered by stratified squamous non-keratinised epithelium which dips into the underlying tissue to form crypts. The lymphocytes lie beneath the epithelium and on the sides of the crypts. These are collected to form nodules. "T lymphocytes" are present in the perifollicular area.

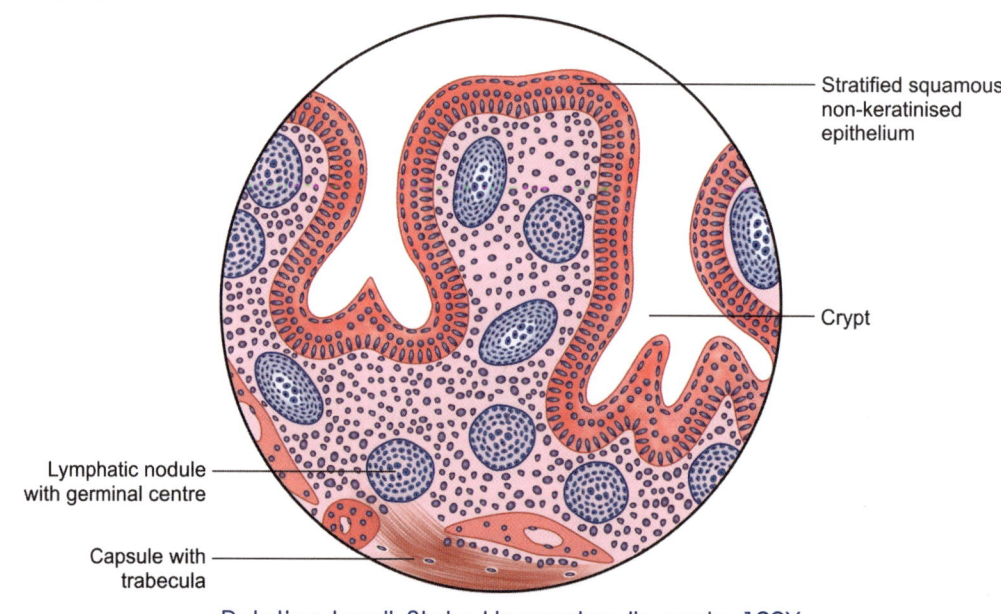

Stratified squamous non-keratinised epithelium

Crypt

Lymphatic nodule with germinal centre

Capsule with trabecula

Palatine tonsil. Stain: Haematoxylin-eosin, 100X

Thymus

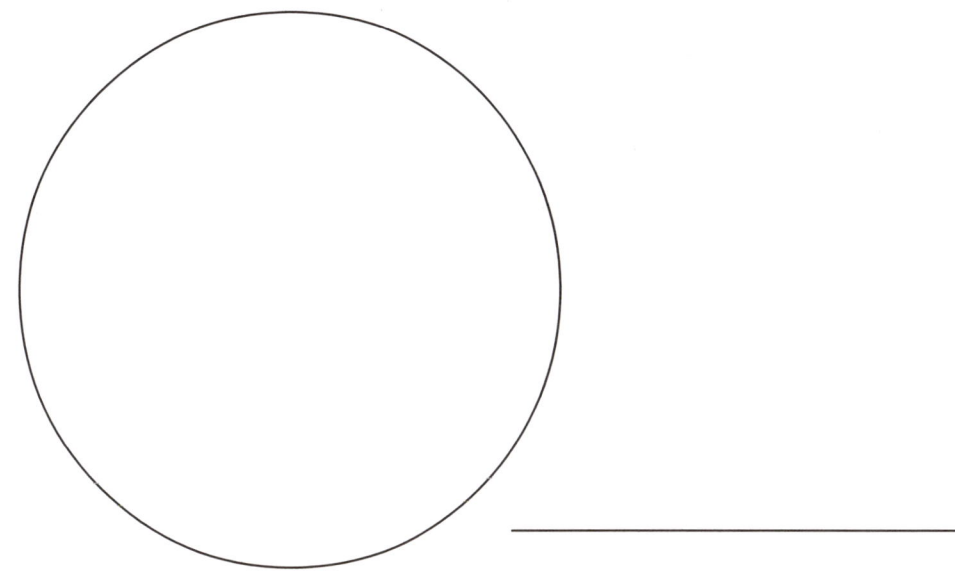

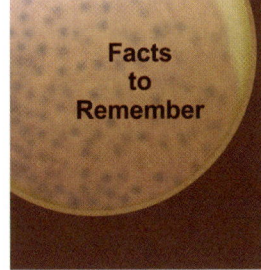

Facts to Remember

Palatine Tonsil

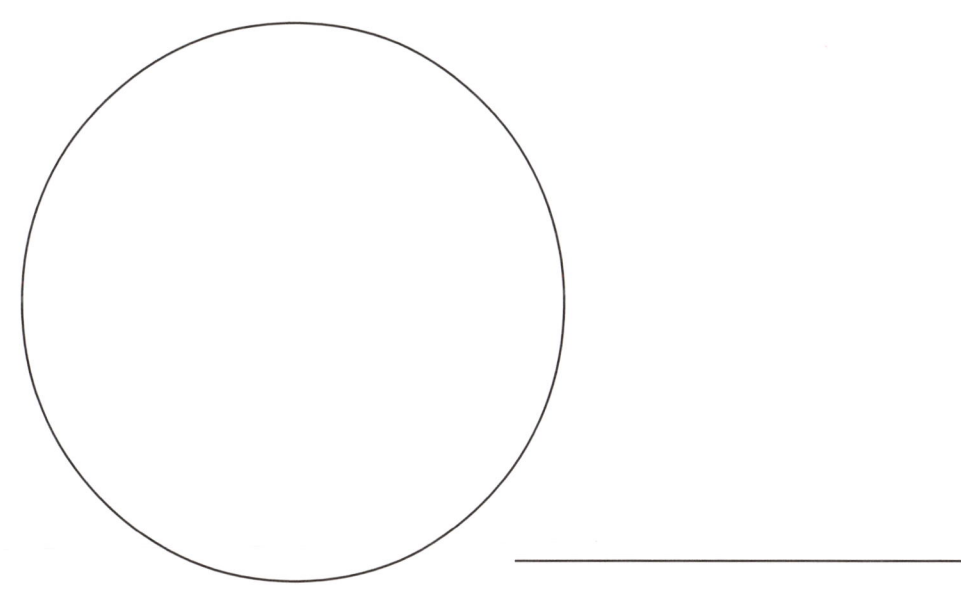

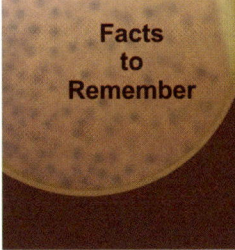

Facts to Remember

9. The Glands

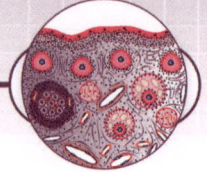

The glands are classified as endocrine and exocrine glands. Salivary glands are exocrine in nature.

SALIVARY GLANDS

Three pairs of salivary glands secrete saliva which is poured into the oral cavity. These are: (i) Parotid gland—serous; (ii) submandibular gland—mixed and predominantly serous; (iii) sublingual gland—mucus.

Parotid Gland

Each acinus is rounded and is lined by pyramidal cells surrounding a very small lumen.

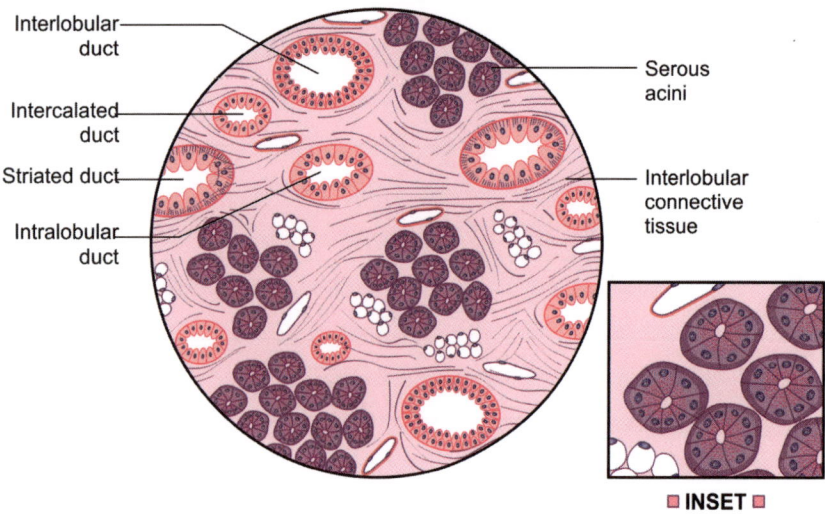

Parotid gland. Stain: Haematoxylin-eosin, 400X

Submandibular Gland

This glands consist of both serous and mucous acini. The mucous acinus is lined by truncated columnar cells. Between mucous cells and the basement membrane are half-moon shaped polyhedral granular serous cells. These cells are known as **demilunes of Giannuzzi**.

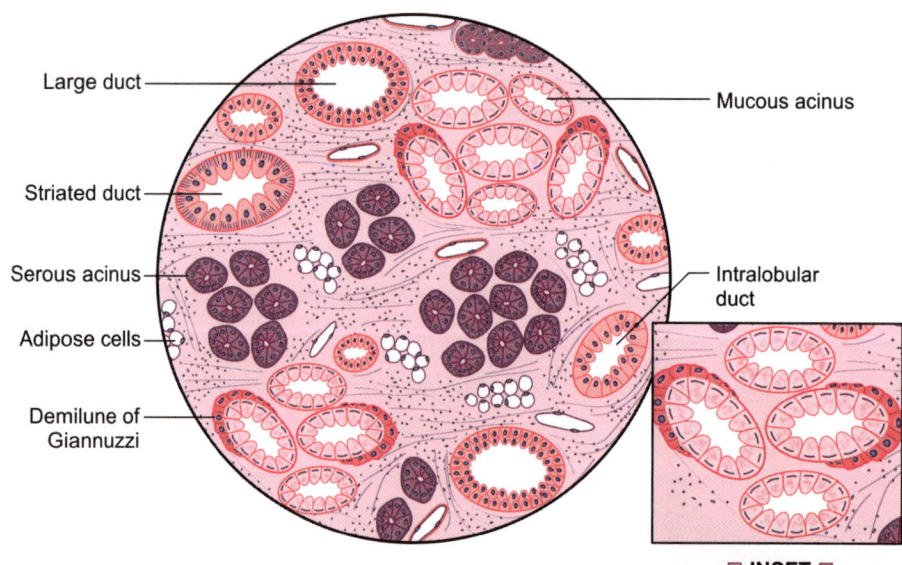

Submandibular gland. Stain: Haematoxylin-eosin, 400X

Parotid Gland

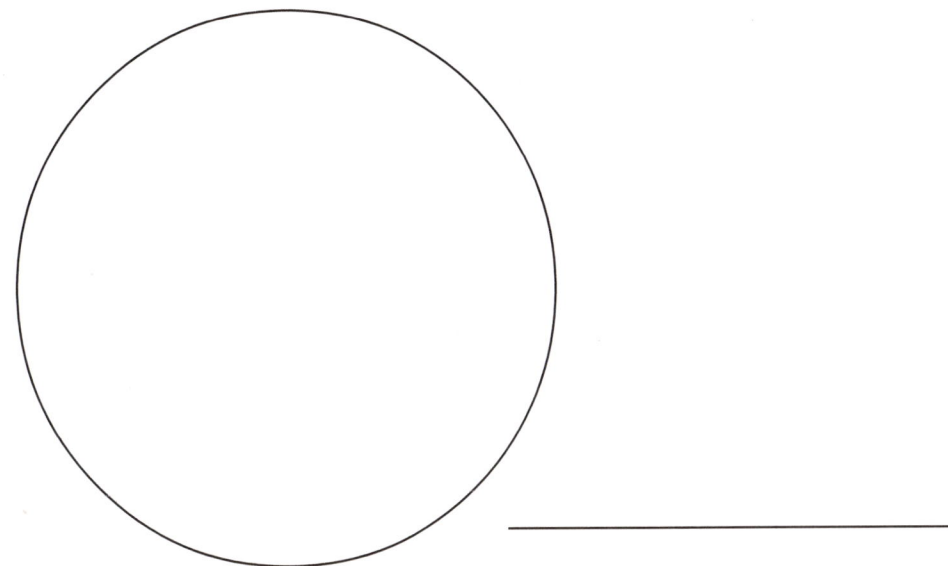

_____

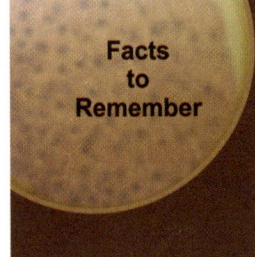

Facts to Remember

_____

_____

_____

Submandibular Gland

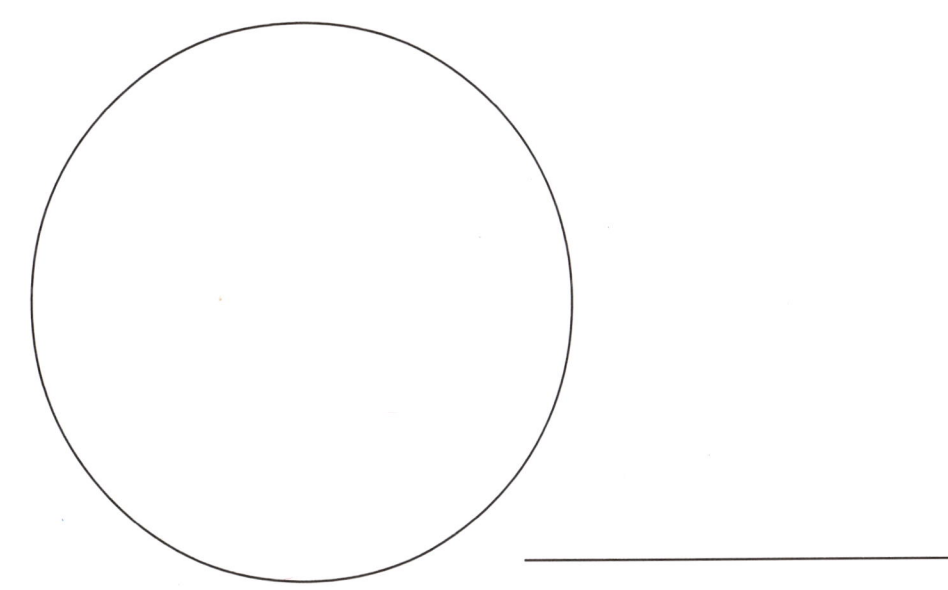

_____

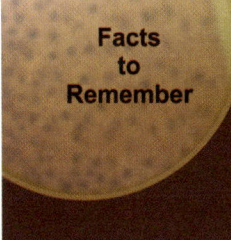

Facts to Remember

_____

_____

_____

Sublingual Gland

These acini are lined by truncated columnar cells as seen by H and E stain. The cytoplasm seems to be vacuolated. Demilunes of Giannuzzi are seen.

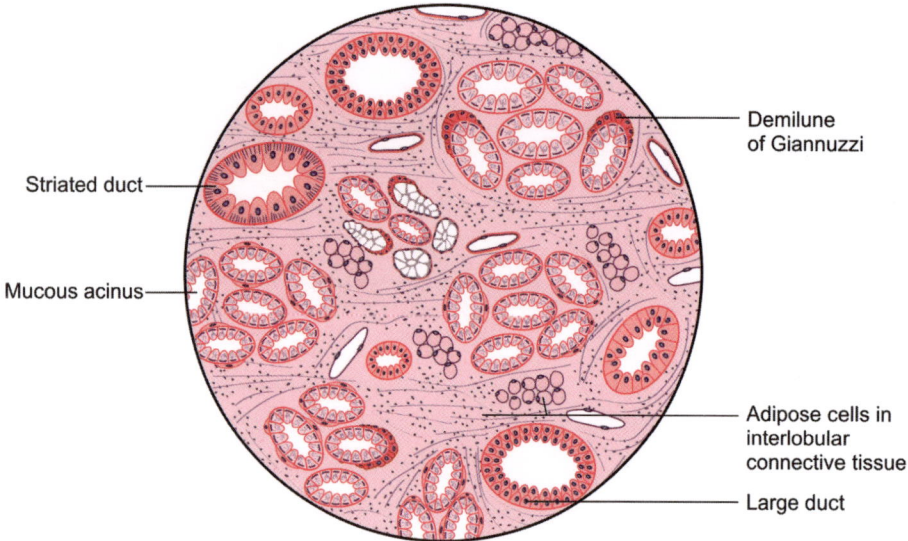

Striated duct

Demilune of Giannuzzi

Mucous acinus

Adipose cells in interlobular connective tissue

Large duct

Sublingual gland. Stain: Haematoxylin-eosin, 400X

VARIOUS TYPES OF GLANDS (diagrammatic)

Sublingual Gland

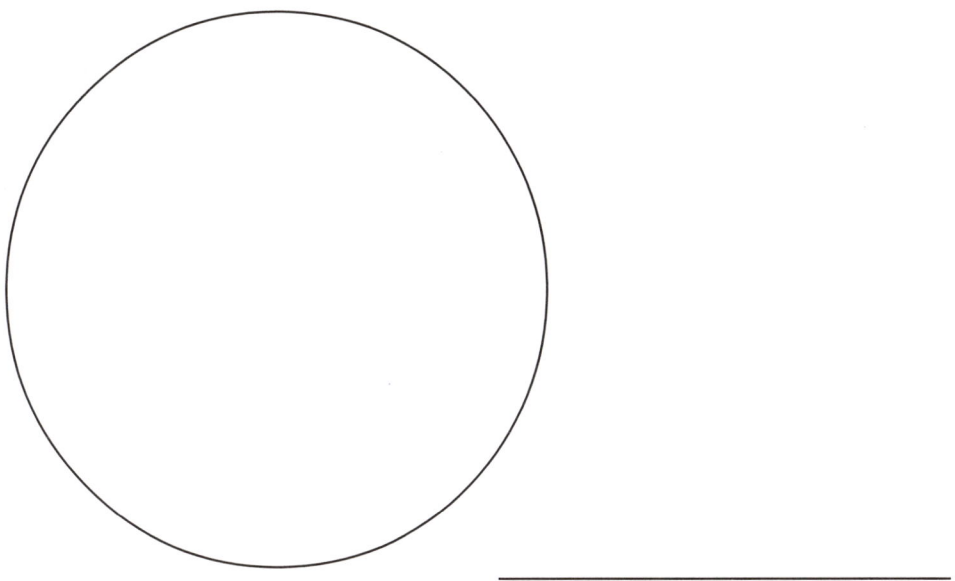

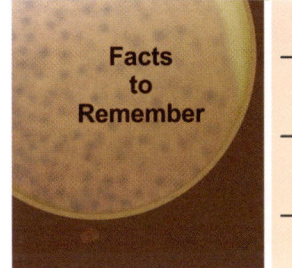

**Facts
to
Remember**

_____

_____

_____

Classification of Glands

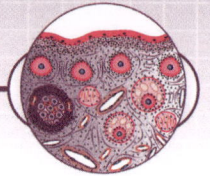

10. Integumentary System

Integumentary system consists of skin and its various appendages. Skin consists of two main layers:

a. _____

b. _____

EPIDERMIS

i. *Stratum basale:* _____
_____

ii. *Stratum spinosum:* _____
_____

iii. *Stratum granulosum:* _____
_____

iv. *Stratum lucidum:* _____
_____

v. *Stratum corneum:* _____
_____

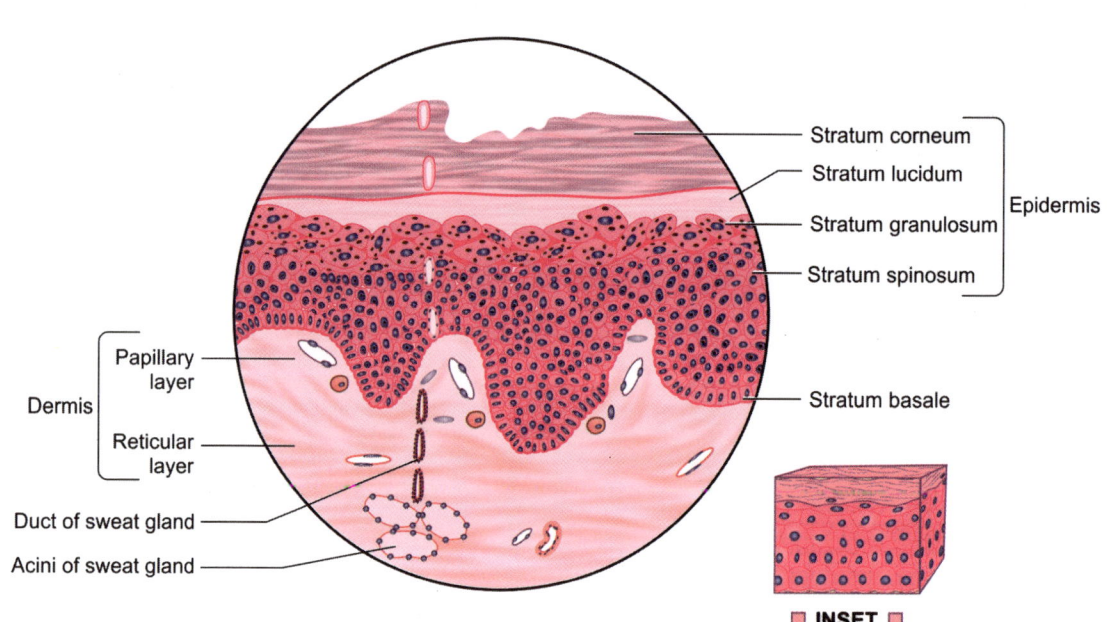

Skin of palm. Stain: Haematoxylin-eosin, 400X

Types of Skin

Thick skin, e.g. skin of palm and sole. The epidermis is very thick especially the stratum corneum. This skin contains numerous sweat glands.

Thin skin, e.g. skin over the rest of the body. Its characteristic features are the presence of hair follicles, sebaceous glands and arrector pili muscles.

Thick Skin

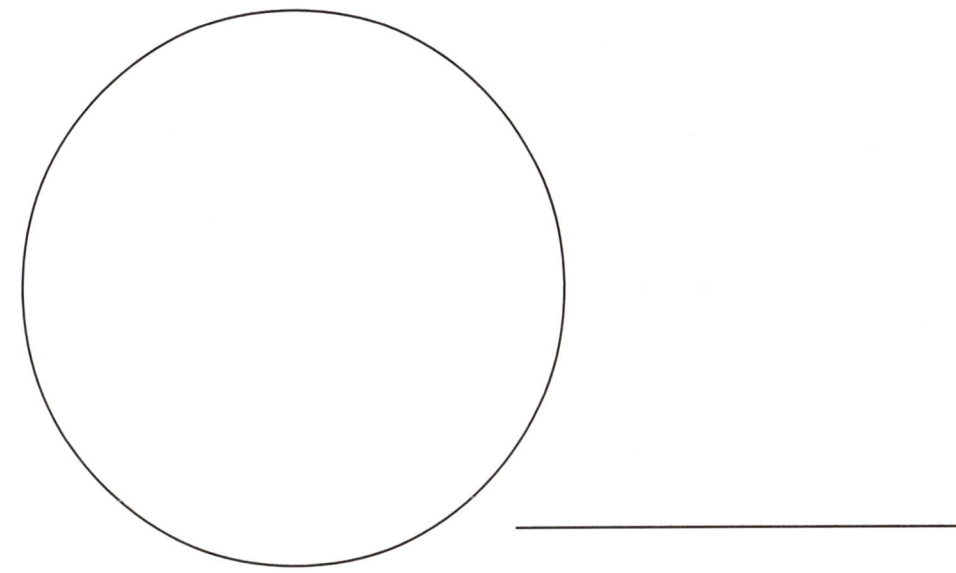

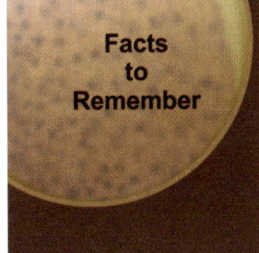

**Facts
to
Remember**

Thin Skin

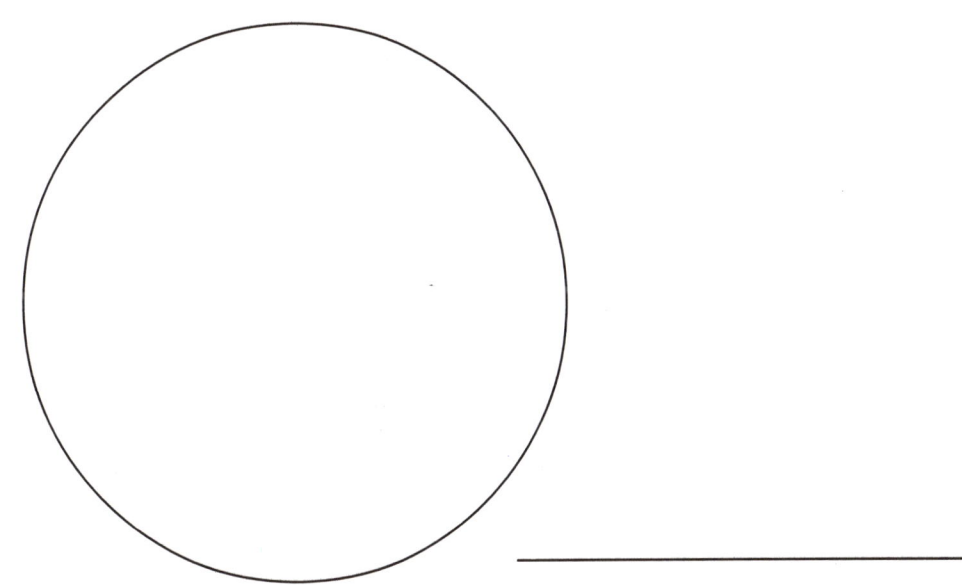

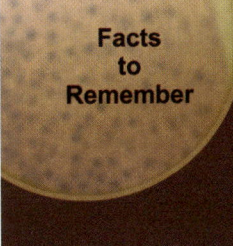

**Facts
to
Remember**

Hair Follicles

Hair follicle comprises the hair root—the part of hair inside the skin and hair shaft, the part protruding beyond the level of epidermis. The hair root is comprised of *medulla*, *cortex* and *cuticle* from within outwards. The hair root is covered by *inner root sheath* derived from stratum corneum. The inner root sheath consists of a cuticle, lying adjacent to cuticle of hair root, Huxley's layer of 2–3 layers of flattened nucleated cells and Henle's layer of single layer of cuboidal cells, from inside out. The *outer root sheath* is comprised of nucleated cells from stratum spinosum and stratum basale. Still outside is the connective tissue sheath.

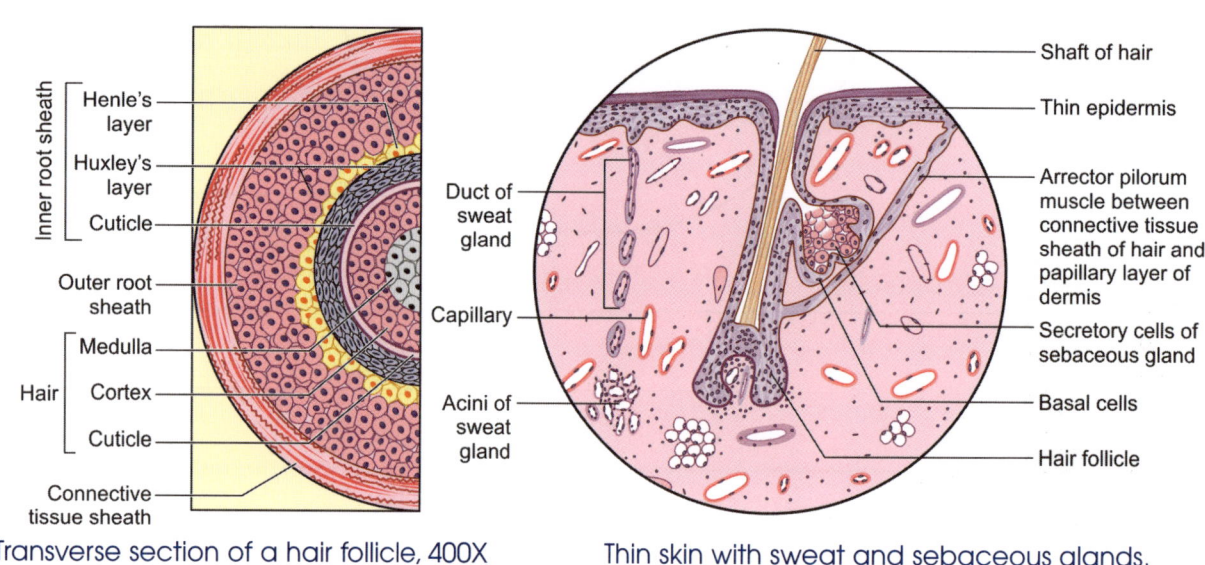

Transverse section of a hair follicle, 400X

Thin skin with sweat and sebaceous glands.
Stain: Haematoxylin-eosin, 100X

Sebaceous Glands

Sebaceous glands are *holocrine* glands and are scattered in the superficial layer of the dermis. These are absent in the palm and sole.

_____

_____

_____

_____

Sweat Gland

_____

_____

_____

_____

_____

Holocrine sebaceous gland

Secretory cells

Basal cells

Hair Follicles

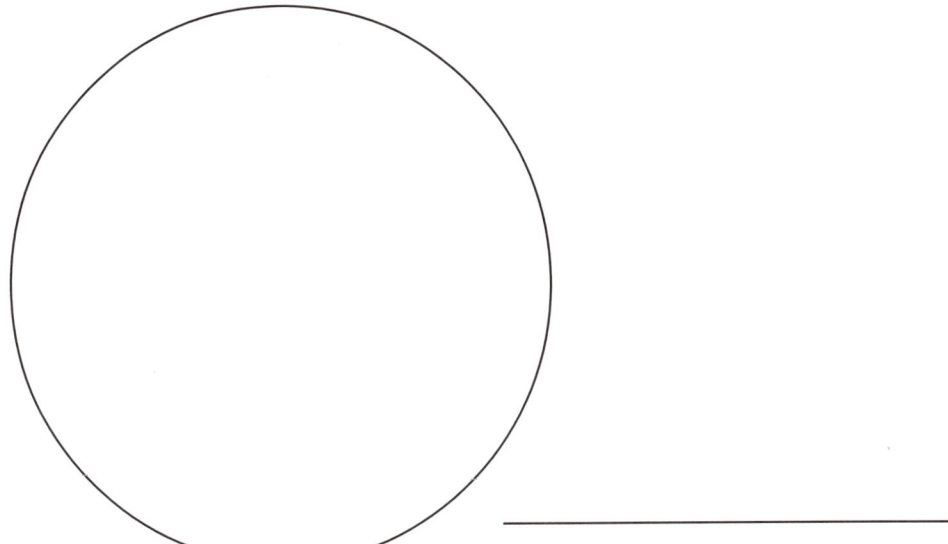

_____

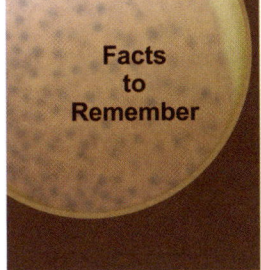
Facts
to
Remember

_____

_____

_____

Sebaceous Glands

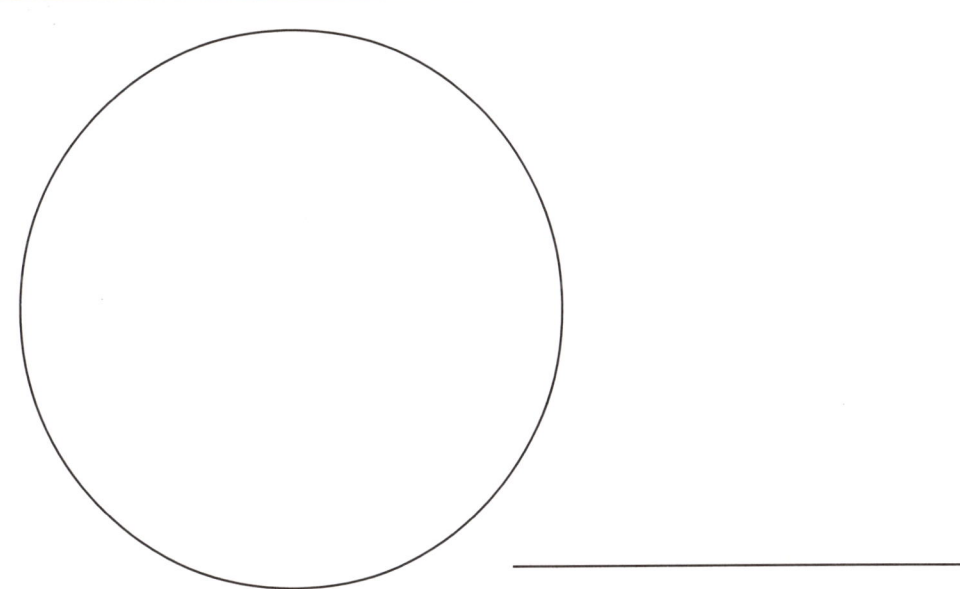

_____

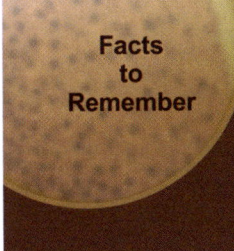
Facts
to
Remember

_____

_____

_____

ADDITIONAL FIGURES/NOTES

ADDITIONAL FIGURES/NOTES

11. Respiratory System

The respiratory system provides for the intake of oxygen and elimination of carbon dioxide. Functionally the respiratory system is divided into:

i. Conducting part which comprises nose, nasopharynx, larynx, trachea and bronchial tree till the level of terminal bronchioles. These are always patent for respiration.

ii. Respiratory part comprising of respiratory bronchioles, alveolar duct, atria, alveolar sac and alveoli. These are present in the spongy part of lung for exchange of gases.

TRACHEA

_____

_____

_____

_____

_____

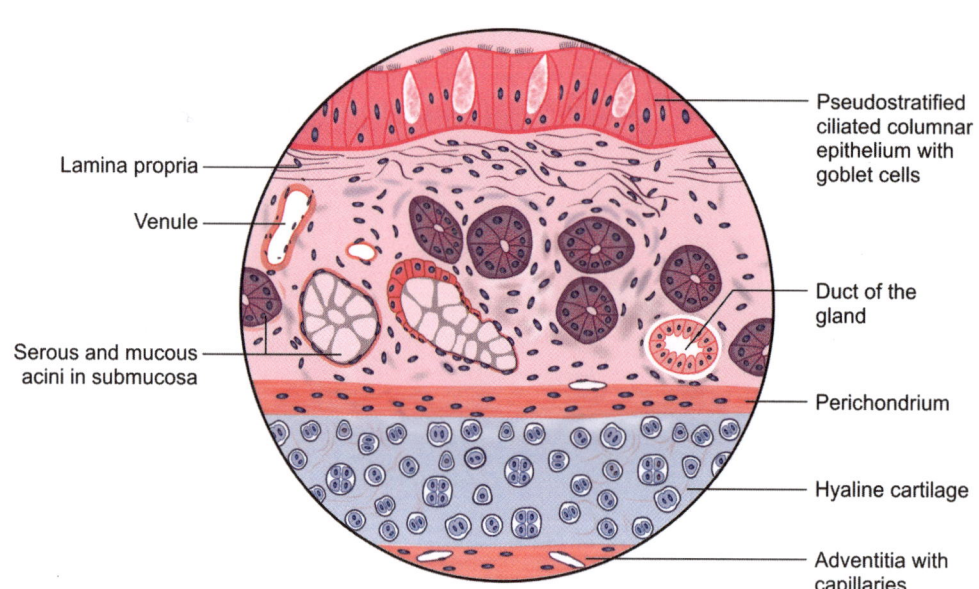

Trachea. Stain: Haematoxylin-eosin, 100X

Labels:
- Pseudostratified ciliated columnar epithelium with goblet cells
- Lamina propria
- Venule
- Duct of the gland
- Serous and mucous acini in submucosa
- Perichondrium
- Hyaline cartilage
- Adventitia with capillaries

BRONCHIAL TUBES

The trachea divides into two *primary bronchi.* Each primary bronchus divides into secondary bronchi which in turn divide into tertiary or segmental bronchi. The tertiary bronchi continue to divide till *terminal bronchioles.*

Each terminal bronchiole continues to divide into 2–4 *respiratory bronchioles*. These break up into 2–10 *alveolar ducts* which give rise to *atria, alveolar sacs* and *alveoli.*

*Intrapulmonary bronchus:*_____

_____

_____

_____

_____

Trachea

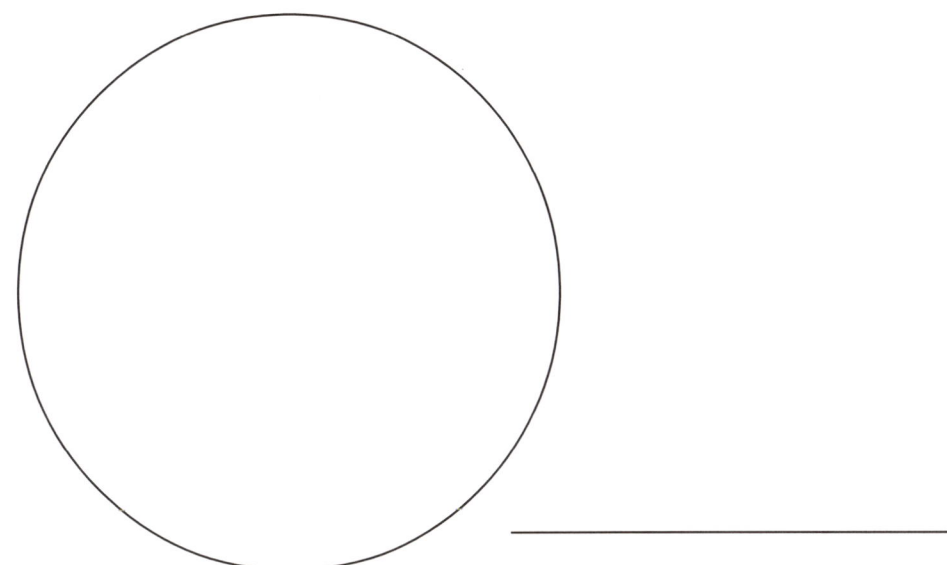

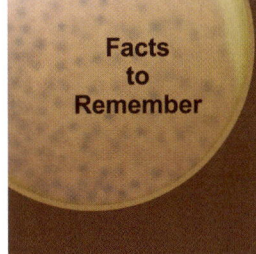

Facts to Remember

Intrapulmonary Bronchus

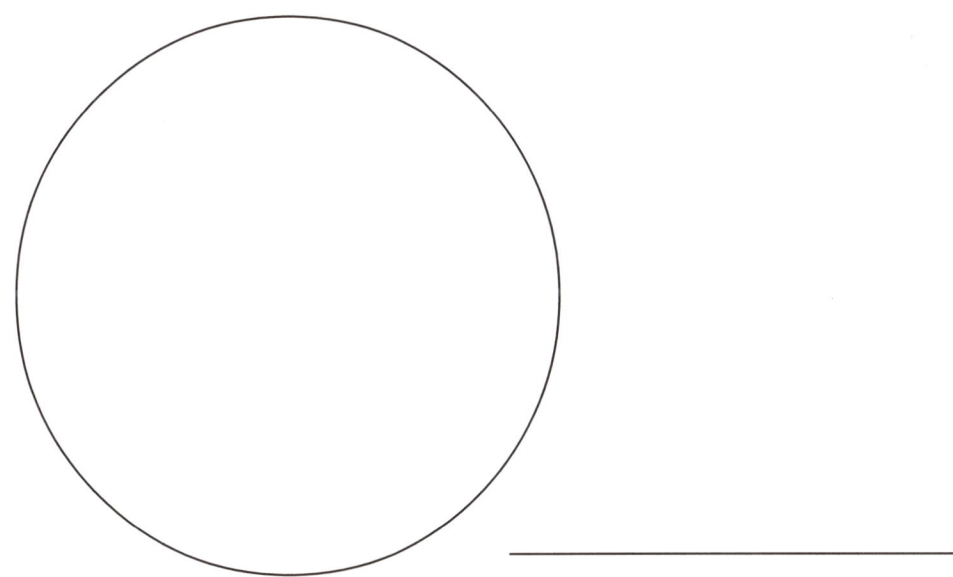

Facts to Remember

Terminal Bronchiole

_____

_____

_____

_____

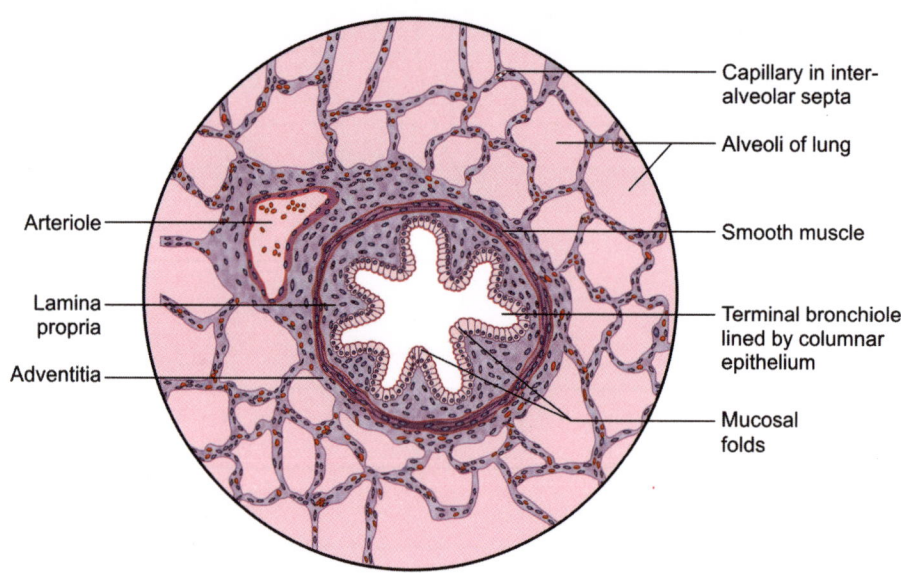

Capillary in inter-alveolar septa

Alveoli of lung

Smooth muscle

Terminal bronchiole lined by columnar epithelium

Mucosal folds

Arteriole

Lamina propria

Adventitia

Terminal bronchiole. Stain: Haematoxylin-eosin, 400X

Alveoli

Alveoli are thin walled polyhedral sacs. The alveoli are lined by two types of cells. Majority of cells lining the alveoli are the *squamous cells* or *type I pneumocytes.* A few are larger cells or *type II pneumocytes.*

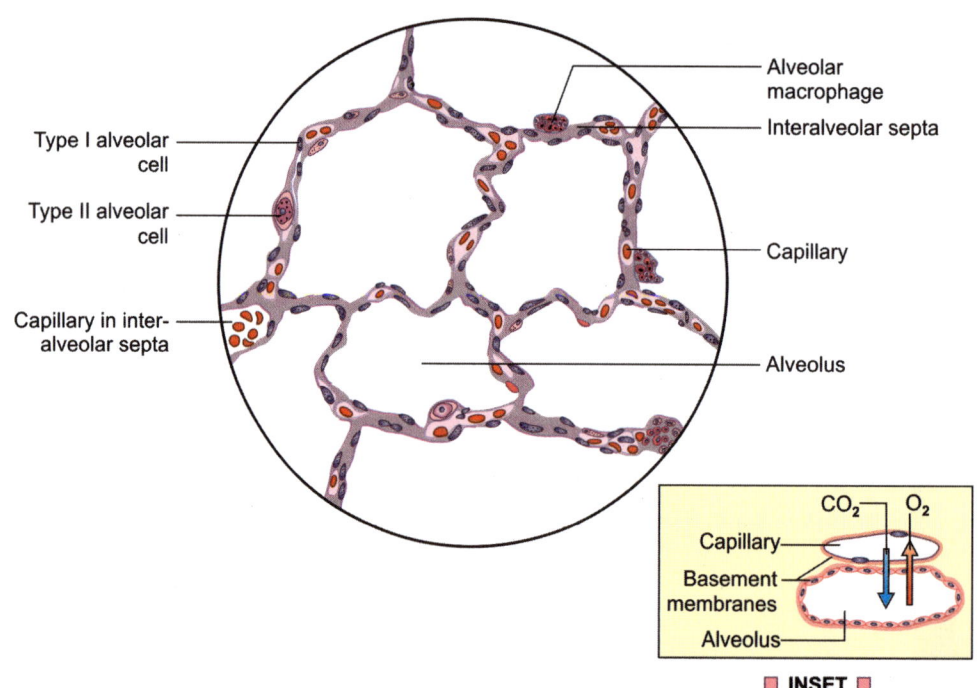

Type I alveolar cell

Type II alveolar cell

Capillary in inter-alveolar septa

Alveolar macrophage

Interalveolar septa

Capillary

Alveolus

CO_2 O_2

Capillary

Basement membranes

Alveolus

■ INSET ■

Alveoli and blood air barrier. Stain: Haematoxylin-eosin, 400X

Terminal Bronchiole

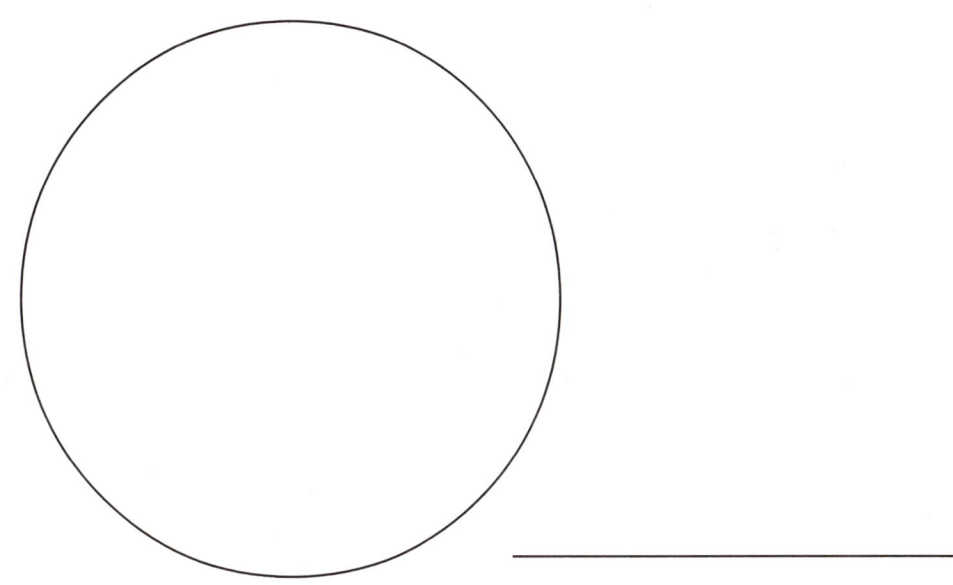

Facts
to
Remember

Alveoli, Interalveolar Septa

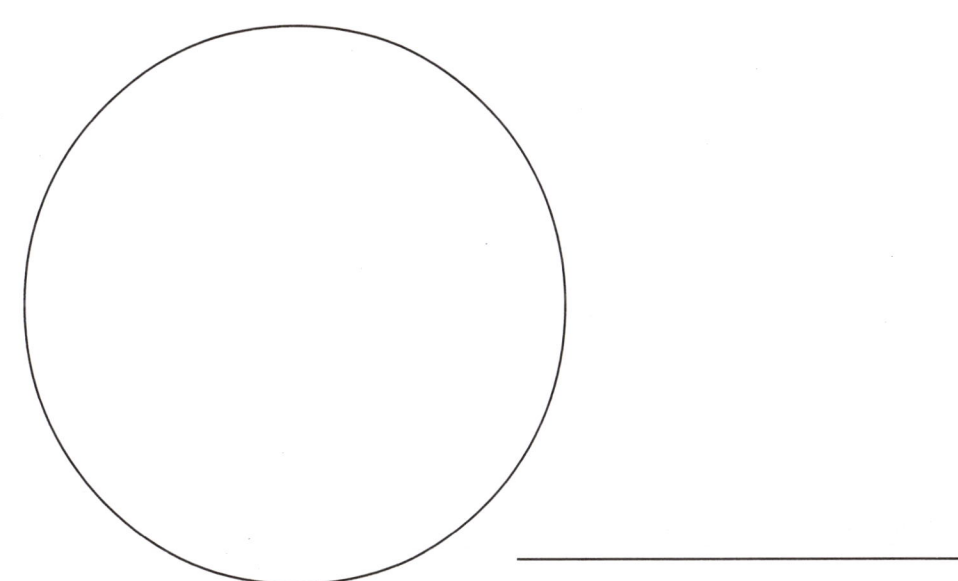

Facts
to
Remember

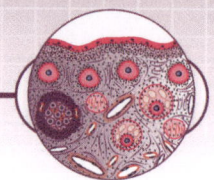

12. Digestive System: Oesophagus and Stomach

*The **digestive system** consists of digestive tract:* (i) Oral cavity/mouth cavity, oesophagus, stomach, small and large intestines including rectum and anal canal, and its associated glands; (ii) salivary glands, liver, gall bladder and pancreas.

General plan of gastrointestinal tract: The wall of the gastrointestinal tract (GIT) from oesophagus to anal canal is made up of the following four layers. 1. Mucous membrane consists of three layers: (a) Epithelium resting on a basement membrane; (b) lamina propria; (c) muscularis mucosae, 2. submucosa, 3. muscularis externa and 4. serosa or adventitia.

Oesophagus

Mucous membrane: _____

_____

_____

Submucosa: _____

Muscularis externa: _____

Adventitia: _____

Oesophagus. Stain: Haematoxylin-eosin, 100X

Labels: Stratified squamous non-keratinised epithelium; Muscularis mucosae; Mucous acini in submucosa; Muscularis externa; Tunica adventitia; Arteriole

Cardio-oesophageal Junction

Mucous membrane: _____

_____

_____

Submucosa: _____

Muscularis externa: _____

Serosa: _____

Oesophagus

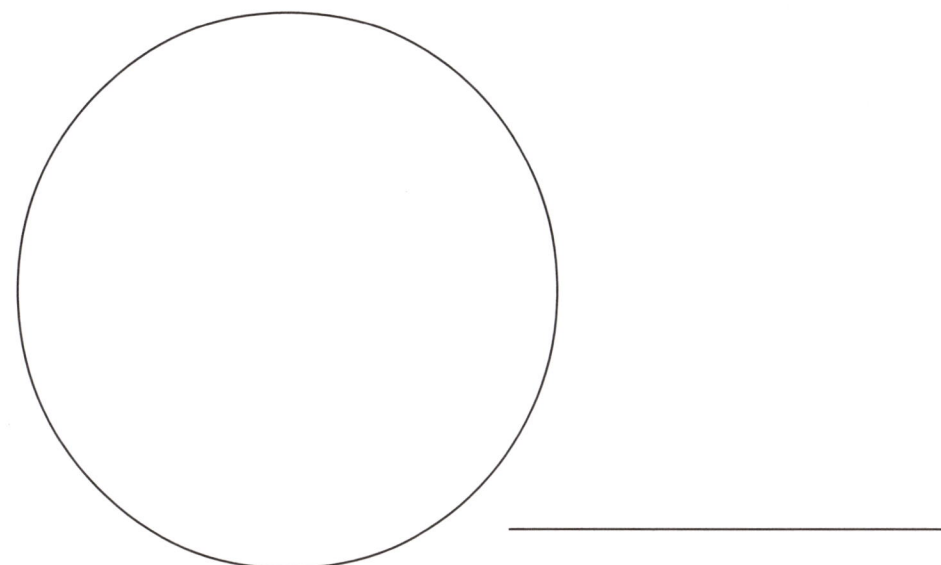

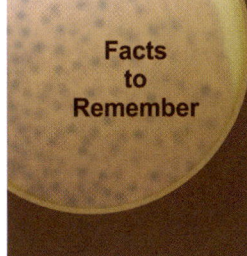

Facts to Remember

_____

_____

_____

Cardio-oesophageal Junction

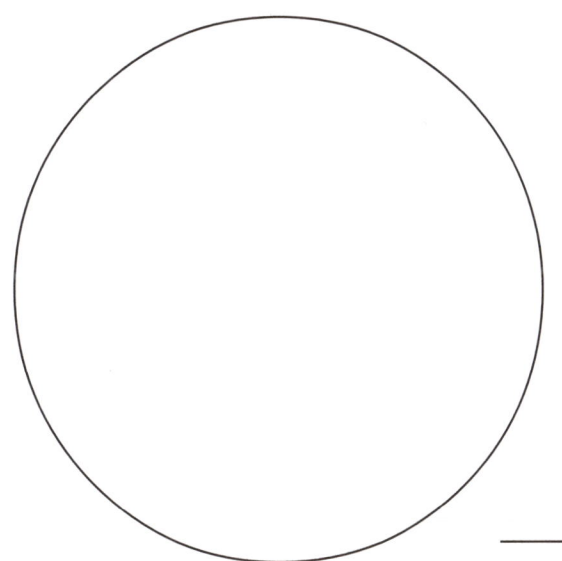

Facts to Remember

_____

_____

_____

Fundus and Body of Stomach

_____

_____

_____

_____

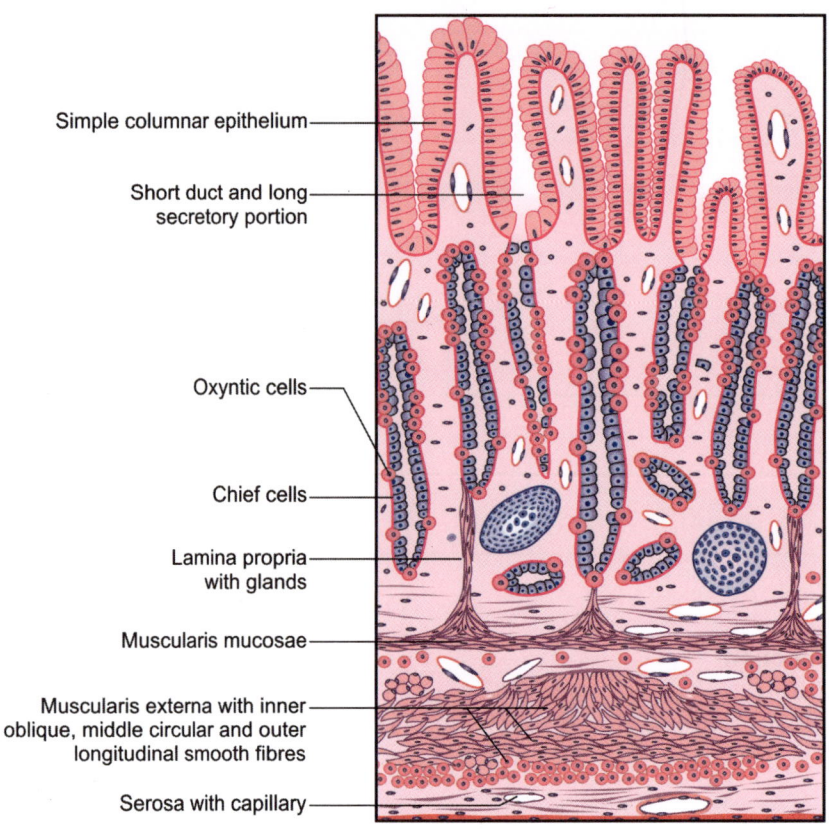

Simple columnar epithelium

Short duct and long
secretory portion

Oxyntic cells

Chief cells

Lamina propria
with glands

Muscularis mucosae

Muscularis externa with inner
oblique, middle circular and outer
longitudinal smooth fibres

Serosa with capillary

Fundus and body of stomach. Stain: Haematoxylin-eosin, 100X

Pyloric Part of Stomach

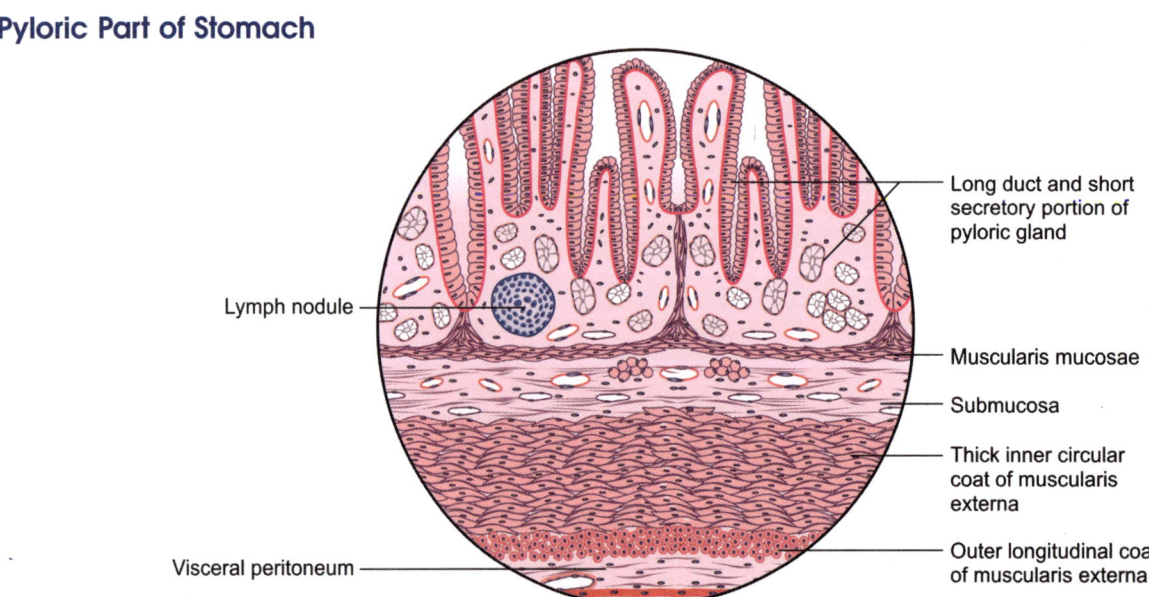

Long duct and short
secretory portion of
pyloric gland

Lymph nodule

Muscularis mucosae

Submucosa

Thick inner circular
coat of muscularis
externa

Outer longitudinal coat
of muscularis externa

Visceral peritoneum

Pyloric part of stomach. Stain: Haematoxylin-eosin, 100X

Fundus and Body of Stomach

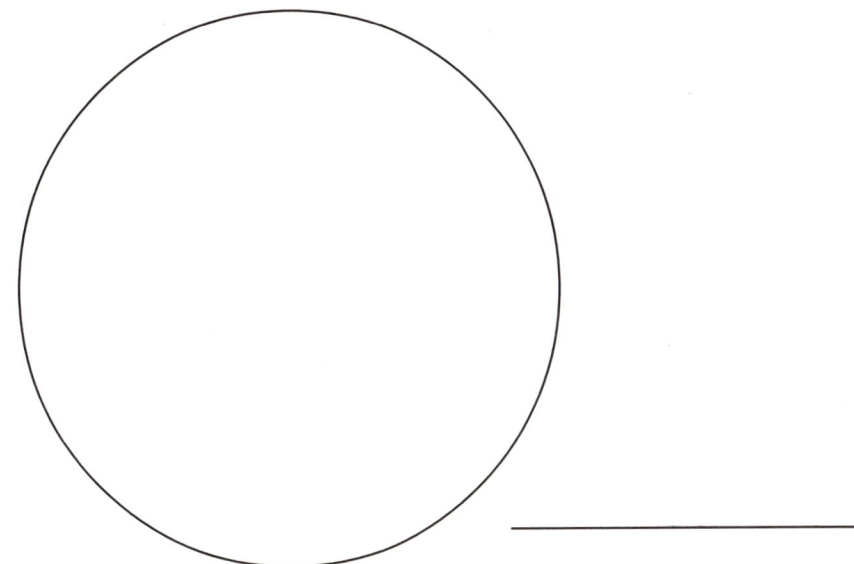

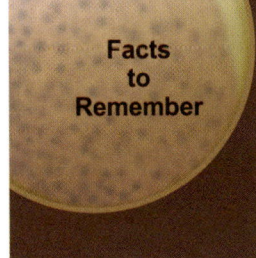

Facts to Remember

_____

_____

_____

Pyloric Part of Stomach

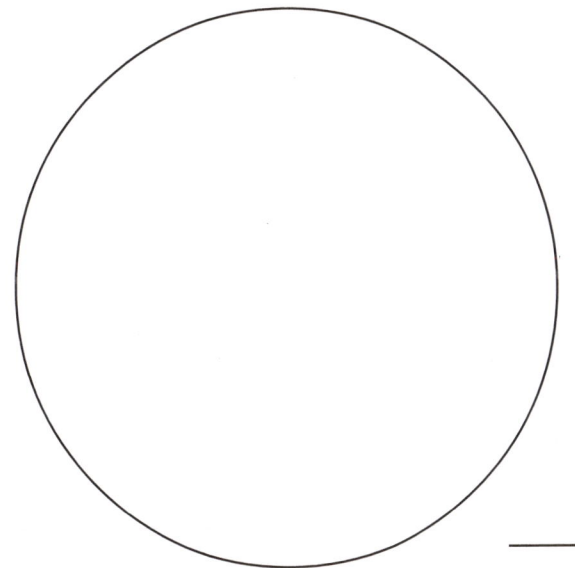

Facts to Remember

_____

_____

_____

13. Digestive System: Small and Large Intestines

GENERAL PLAN

The small intestine divisible into three parts—duodenum, jejunum and ileum. The surface area of the small intestine is increased by the formation of permanent circular folds. The epithelium of the mucous membrane is evaginated to form finger like processes, *the villi*. The epithelial cells have striated border or *brush border*. Lamina propria contains fibroblasts, connective tissue fibres, lymphocytes, eosinophils, macrophages, mast cells, non-myelinated nerve fibres, lymph vessels and capillaries. Lymphocytes may be clustered to form follicles. Following figure shows mucous membrane of small intestine.

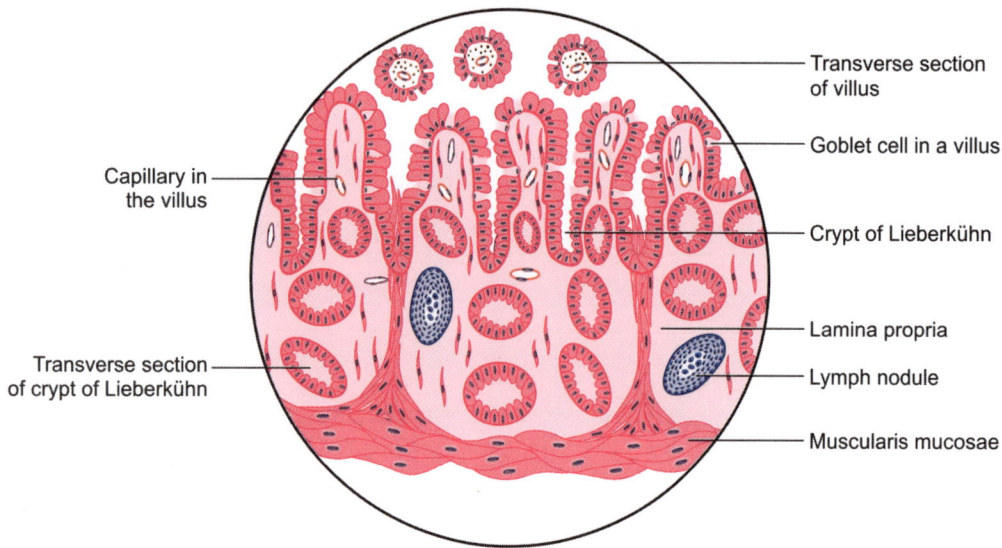

Mucous membrane. Stain: Haematoxylin-eosin, 100X

DUODENUM

_____

_____

_____

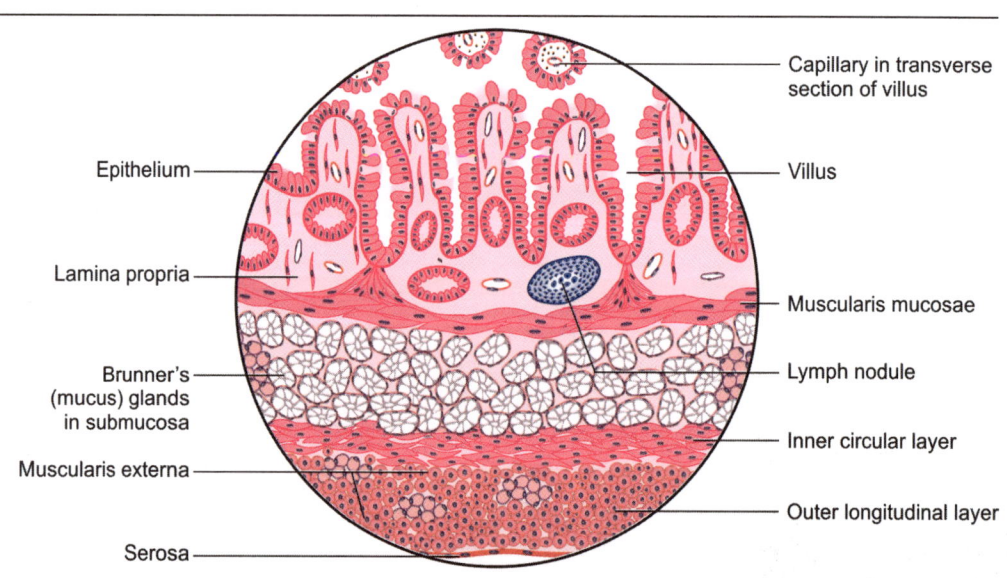

Duodenum. Stain: Haematoxylin-eosin, 100X

Mucous Membrane of Small Intestine

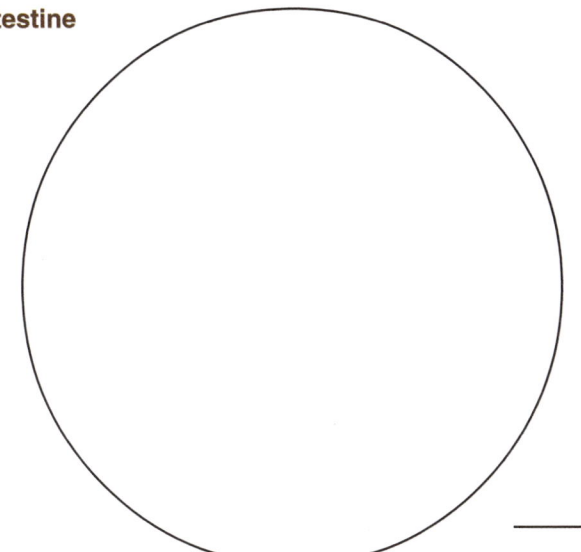

_____

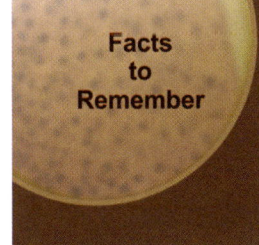

**Facts
to
Remember**

_____

_____

_____

Duodenum

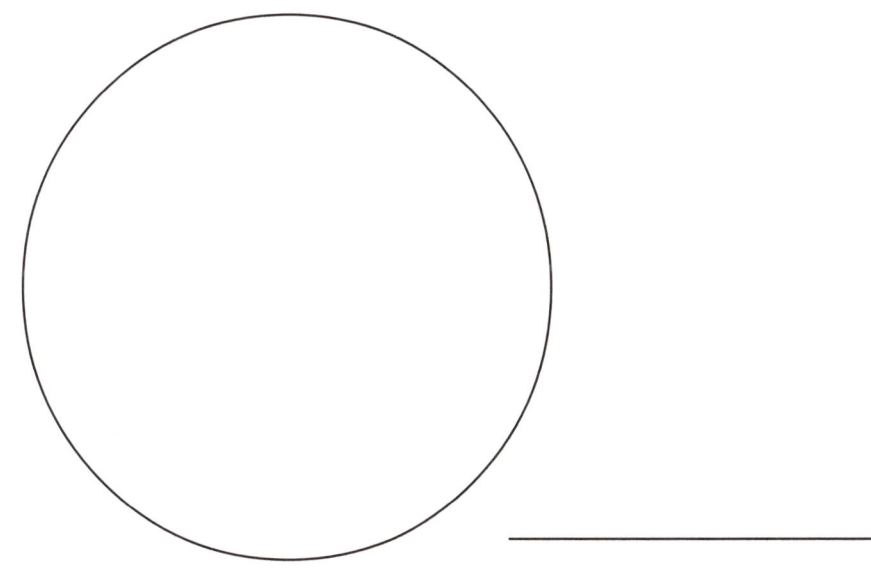

_____

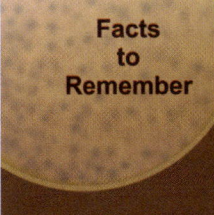

**Facts
to
Remember**

_____

_____

JEJUNUM

_____

_____

_____

_____

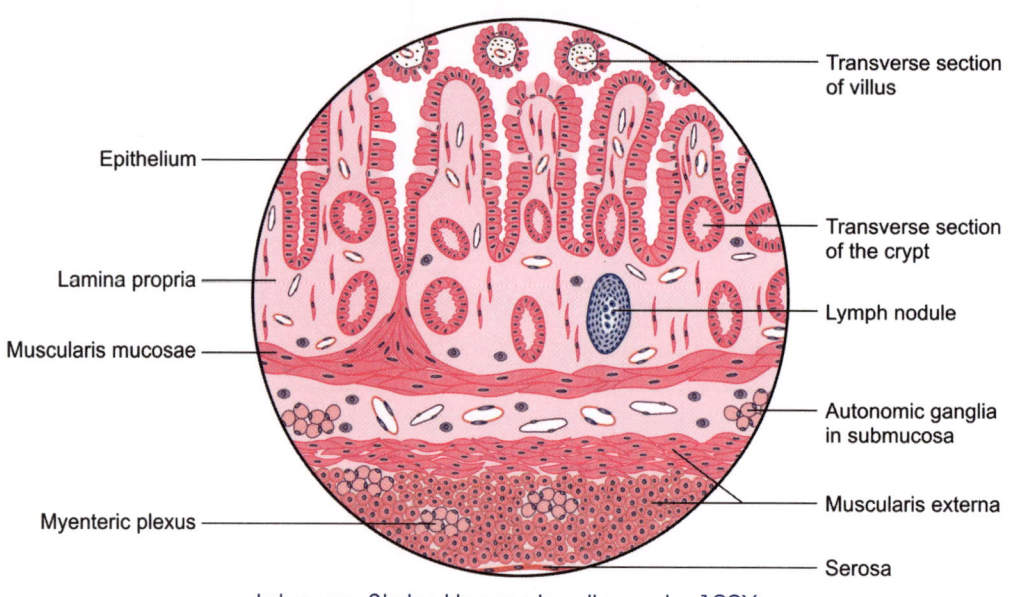

Epithelium

Lamina propria

Muscularis mucosae

Myenteric plexus

Transverse section of villus

Transverse section of the crypt

Lymph nodule

Autonomic ganglia in submucosa

Muscularis externa

Serosa

Jejunum. Stain: Haematoxylin-eosin, 100X

ILEUM

_____

_____

_____

_____

Epithelium

Lamina propria

Lymphoid follicle in lamina propria and submucosa (Peyer's patches)

Muscularis externa

Serosa

Finger shaped villus with goblet cell

Interuptted muscularis mucosae

Submucosa

Myenteric plexus

Ileum. Stain: Haematoxylin-eosin, 100X

Jejunum

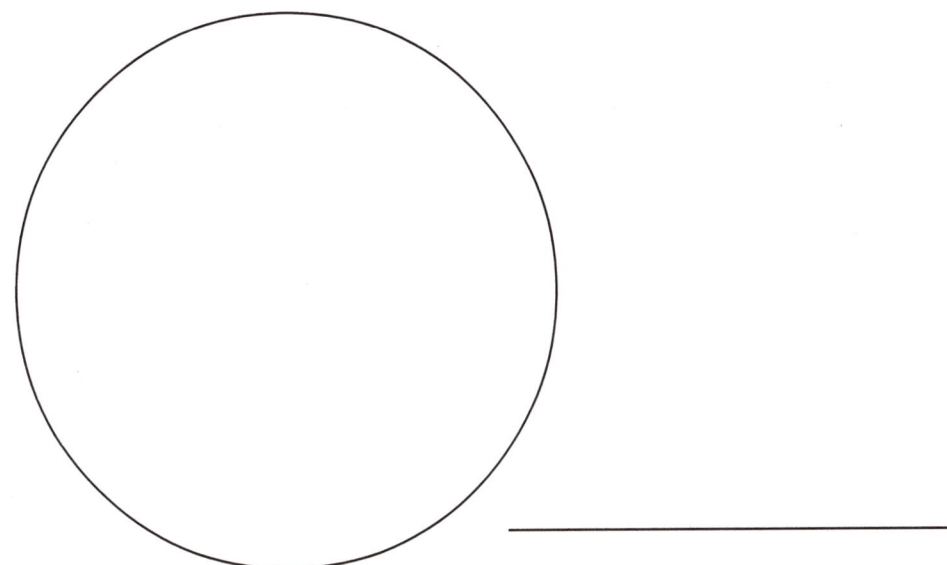

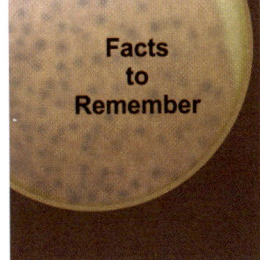

**Facts
to
Remember**

Ileum

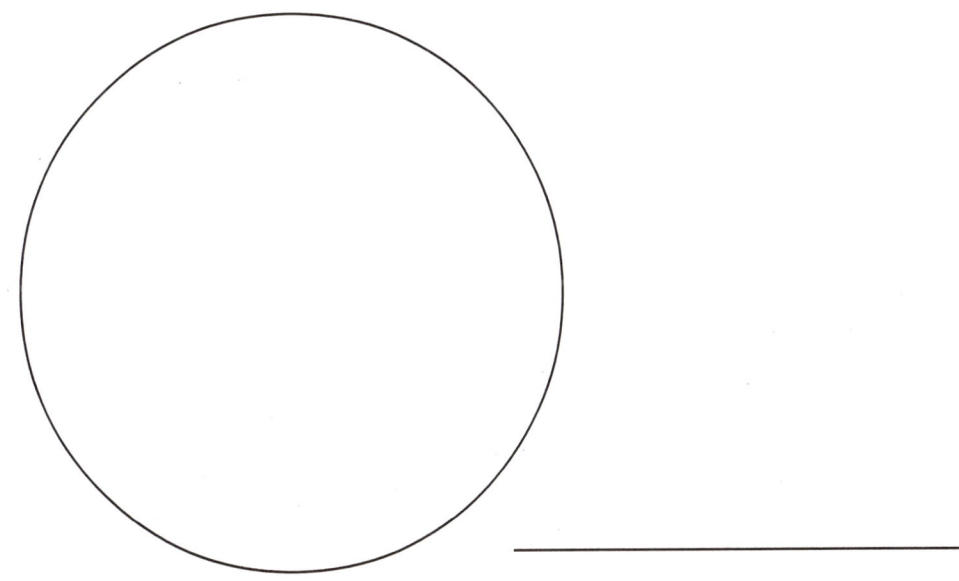

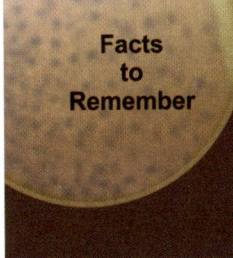

**Facts
to
Remember**

LARGE INTESTINE

The large intestine extends from ileocaecal orifice to the anal orifice. On gross examination, it differs from small intestine in having taenia, sacculations and appendices epiploicae. Histologically the large intestine consists of (i) colon, (ii) vermiform appendix, (iii) rectum and anal canal. Structure of (i) and (ii) is given below:

Colon

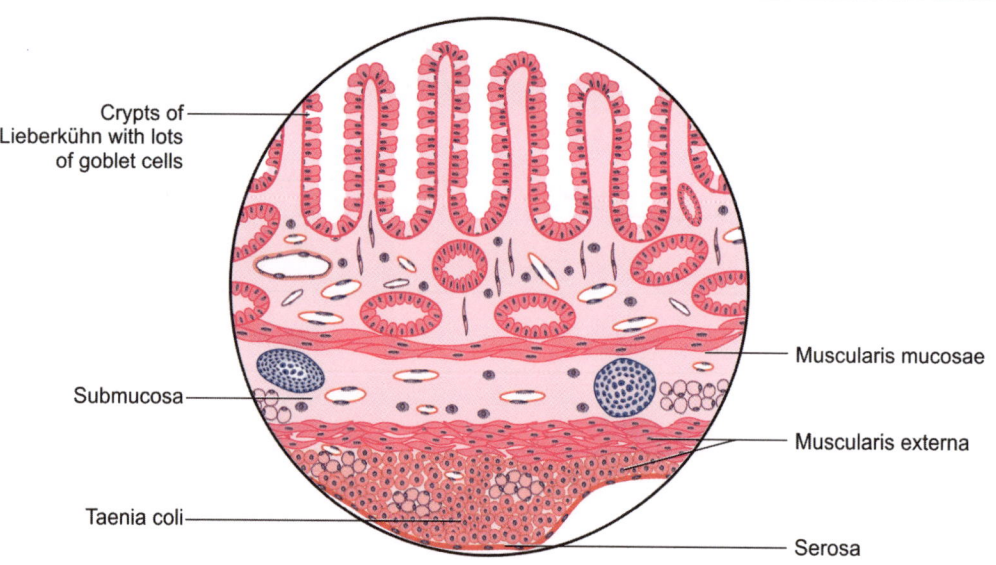

Colon. Stain: Haematoxylin-eosin, 100X

Vermiform Appendix

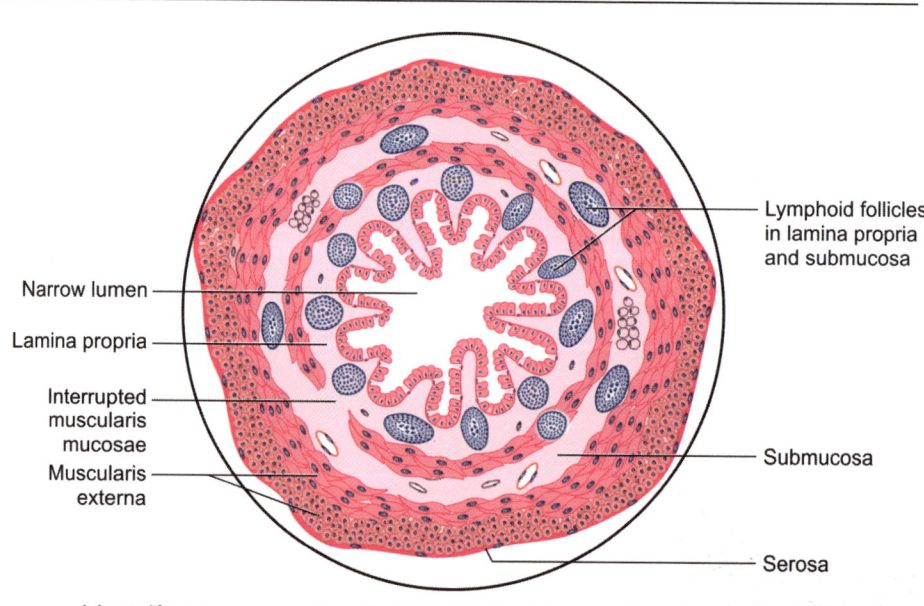

Vermiform appendix of child. Stain: Haematoxylin-eosin, 100X

Colon

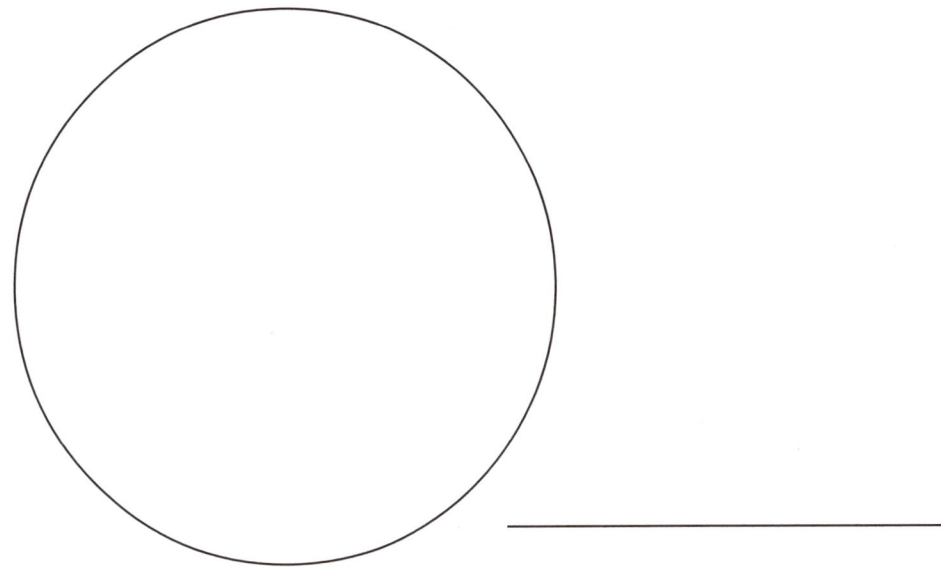

_____

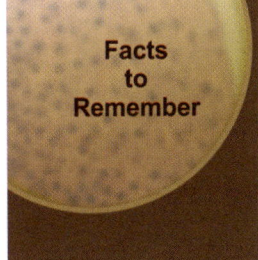

**Facts
to
Remember**

_____

_____

_____

Vermiform Appendix

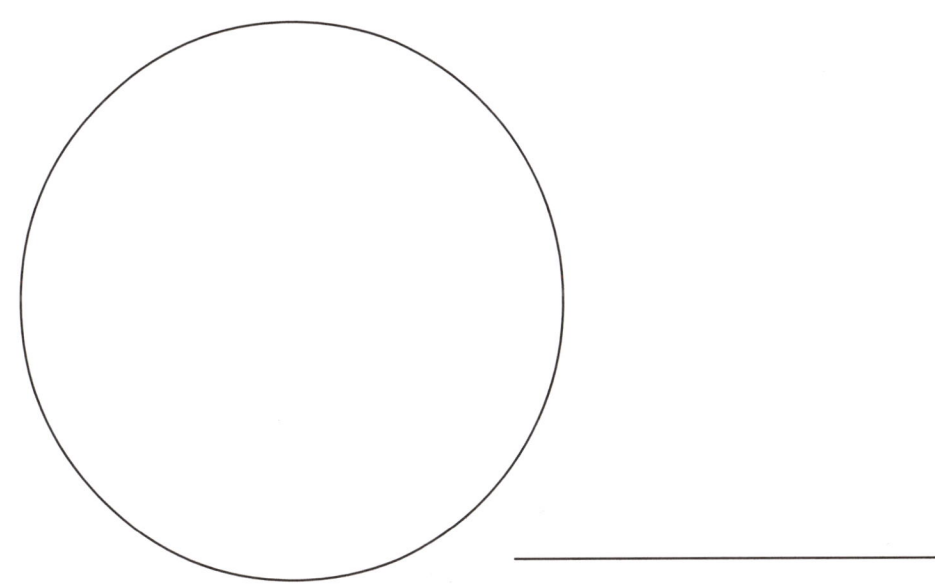

_____

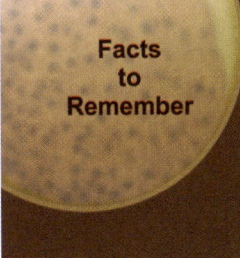

**Facts
to
Remember**

_____

_____

_____

ADDITIONAL FIGURES/NOTES

ADDITIONAL FIGURES/NOTES

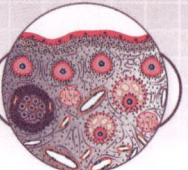

14. Liver, Gall Bladder and Pancreas

LIVER

The liver is the largest gland in the body. Liver comprises numerous, hepatic lobules.

Hepatic Lobule

_____

_____

_____

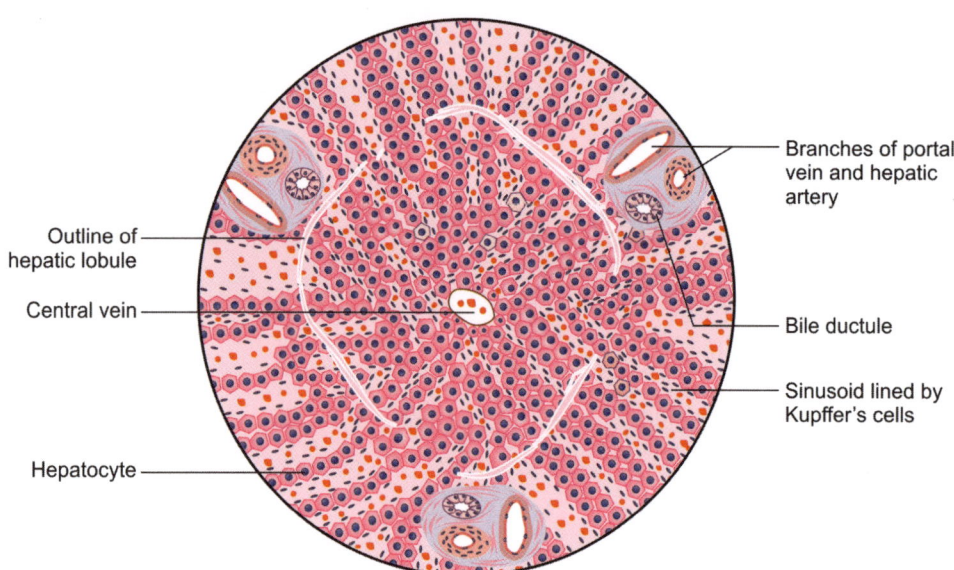

Outline of hepatic lobule

Central vein

Hepatocyte

Branches of portal vein and hepatic artery

Bile ductule

Sinusoid lined by Kupffer's cells

Hepatic lobule. Stain: Haematoxylin-eosin, 400X

Portal Lobule

In man, the connective tissue is sparse and the lobular investment is incomplete. It is apparent mainly at points where three hepatic lobules meet and is known as the *portal lobule*. The portal lobule is triangular to polygonal in shape with portal tract in the centre and three neighbouring central veins on each side of it.

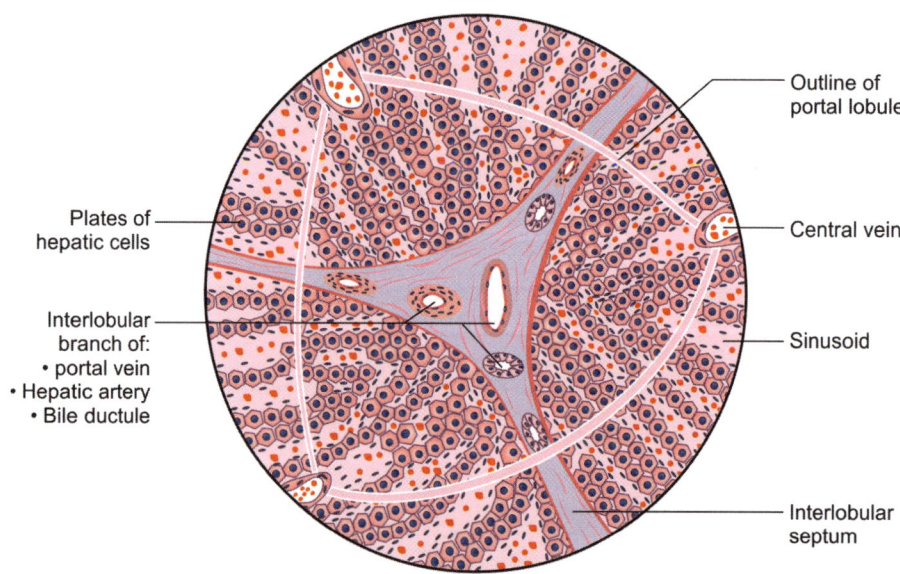

Plates of hepatic cells

Interlobular branch of:
• portal vein
• Hepatic artery
• Bile ductule

Outline of portal lobule

Central vein

Sinusoid

Interlobular septum

Portal lobule. Stain: Haematoxylin-eosin, 400X

Liver, Hepatic Lobule

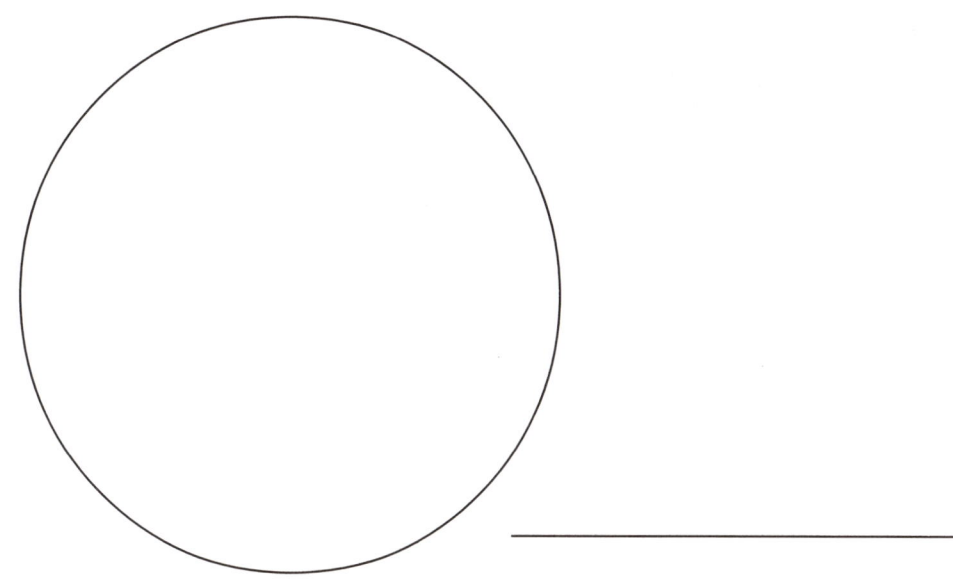

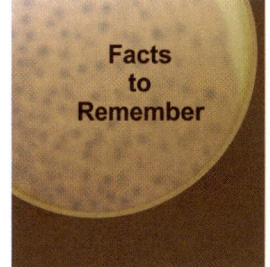

**Facts
to
Remember**

Portal Lobule

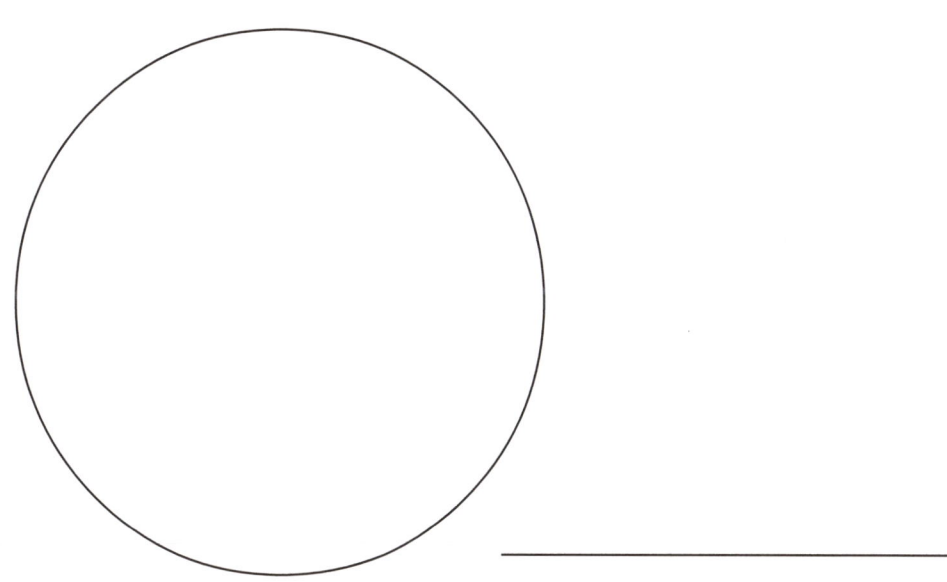

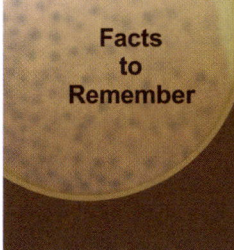

**Facts
to
Remember**

Liver Acinus

The liver acinus is defined as the liver parenchyma around a preterminal branch of hepatic arteriole between two adjacent central veins. The liver sinusoids are lined by reticuloendothelial cells, called Kupffer's cells. Between the hepatic laminae and sinusoid is a potential space called the *space of Disse*. A similar space is present at the portal tract where lymphatics start and is called *space of Mall*.

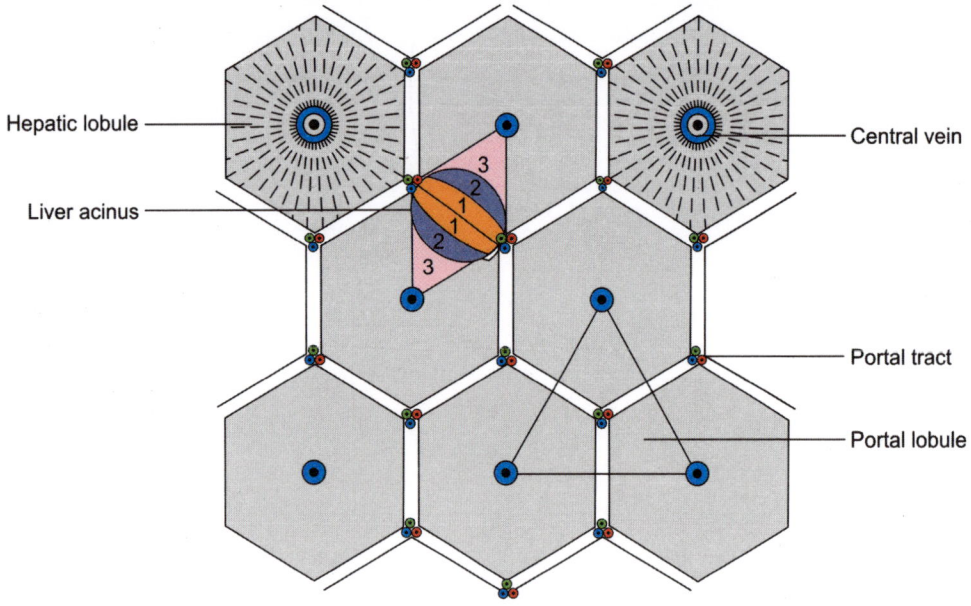

Liver acinus (schematic)

GALL BLADDER

The gall bladder lies on the undersurface of the liver. Its capacity is 30 to 60 millilitres and it concentrates bile to one-tenth of its amount.

_____

_____

_____

_____

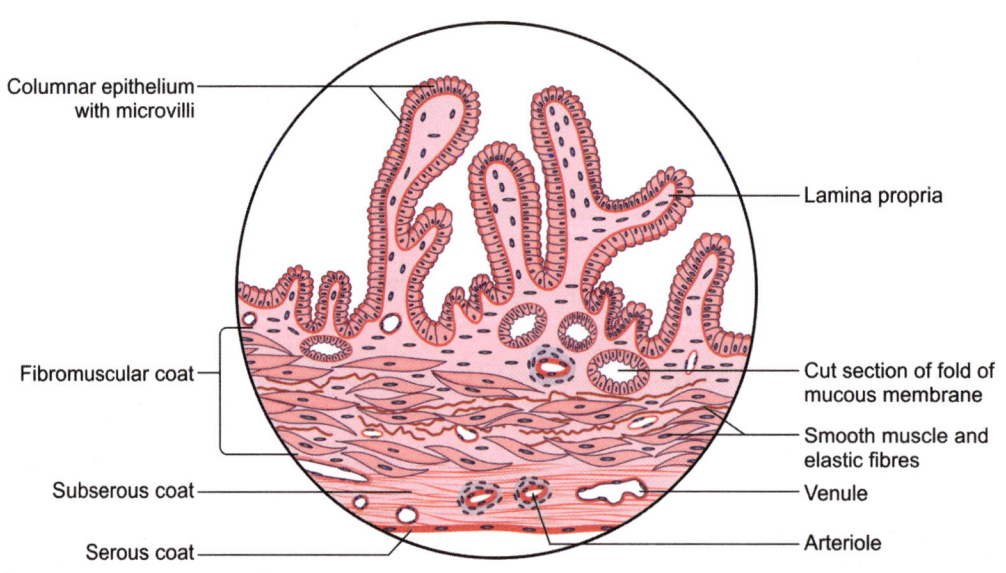

Gall bladder. Stain: Haematoxylin-eosin, 100X

Liver Acinus

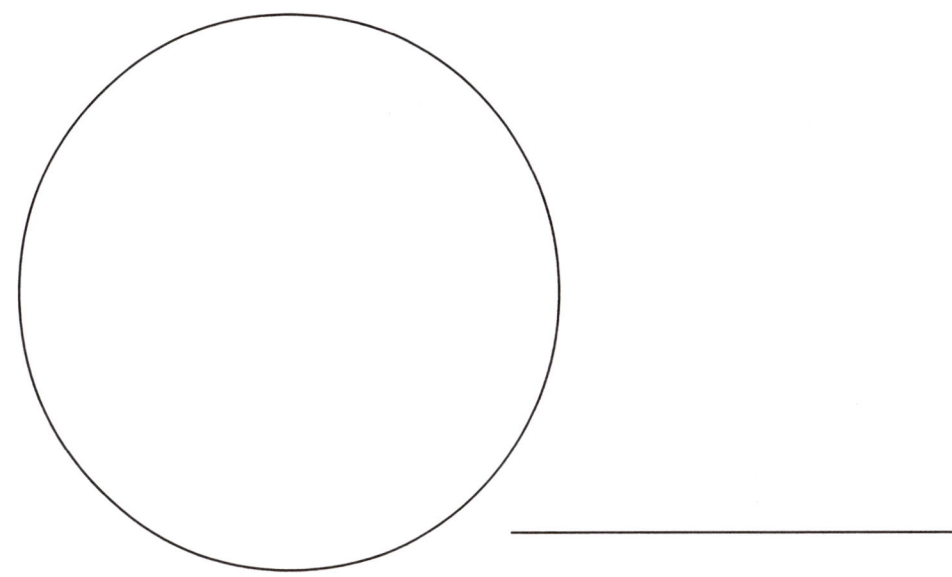

_____

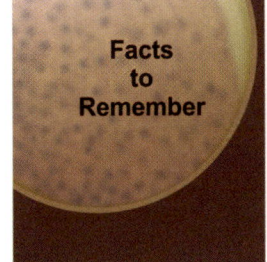

Facts to Remember

_____

_____

_____

Gall Bladder

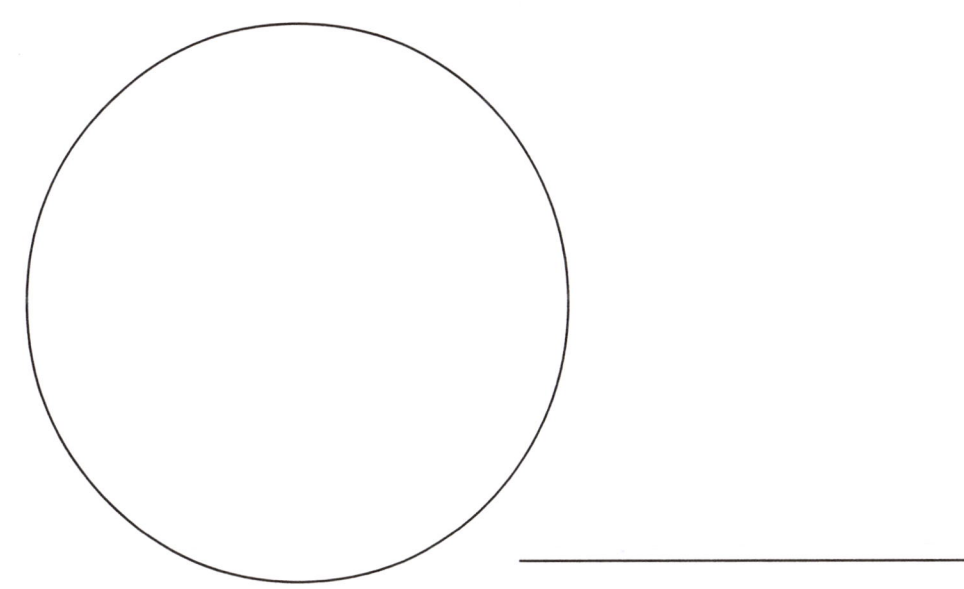

_____

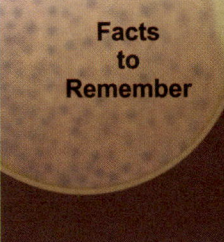

Facts to Remember

_____

_____

_____

PANCREAS

The pancreas is a highly cellular gland composed of an exocrine part secreting pancreatic juice, and an endocrine part called islets of Langerhans, secreting insulin and glucagon. It is made up of:

_____

_____

_____

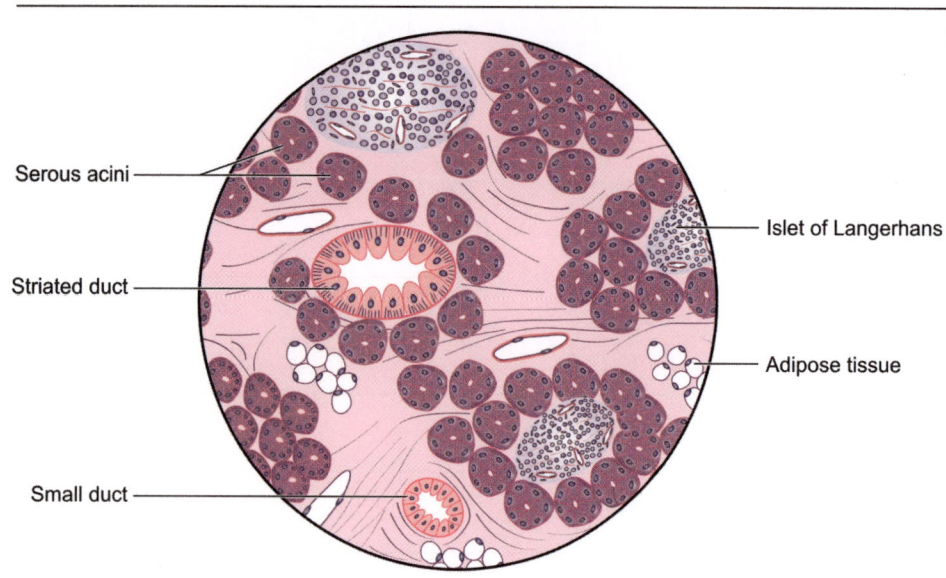

Serous acini

Striated duct

Small duct

Islet of Langerhans

Adipose tissue

Pancreas. Stain: Haematoxylin-eosin, 400X

Constituents of Pancreas

Various constituents of pancreas are: _____

_____

_____

_____

_____

_____

_____

_____

_____

_____

_____

_____

_____

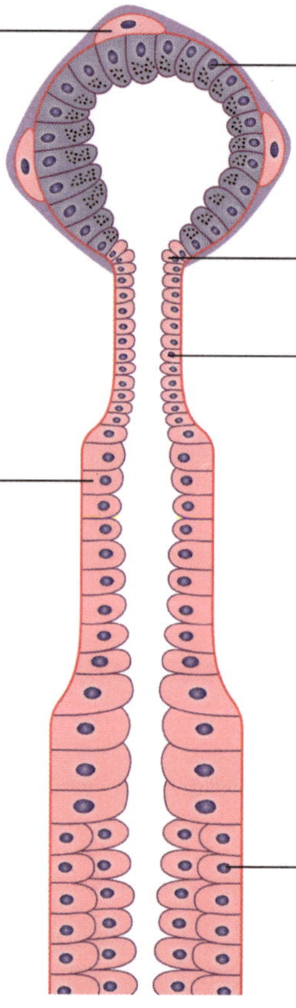

Myoepithelial cell

Acinar cell

Centroacinar cell

Intercalated duct

Interlobular duct

Main pancreatic duct

Stain: Haematoxylin-eosin, 400X

Pancreas

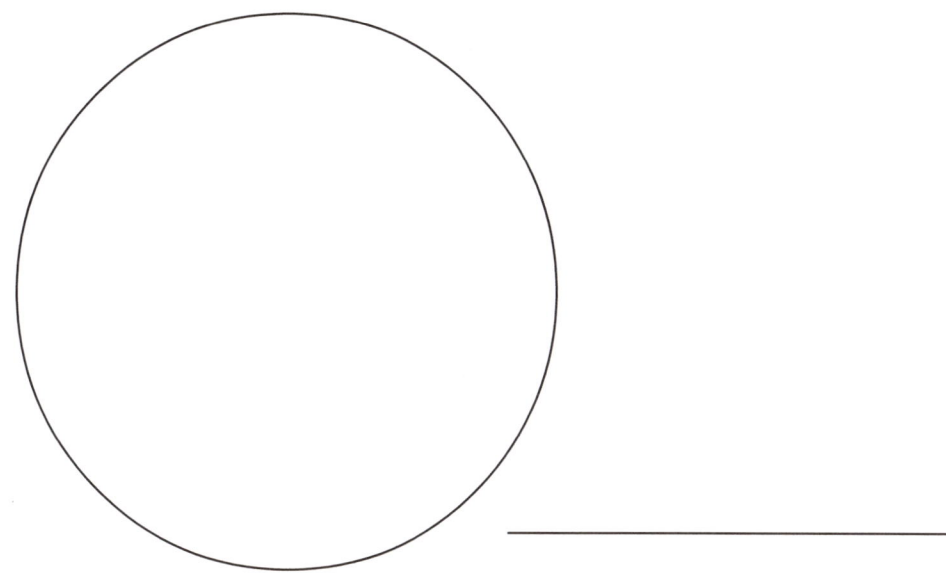

_____

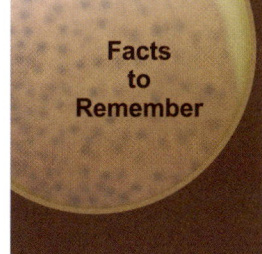

Facts to Remember

_____

_____

_____

Constituents of Pancreas

_____

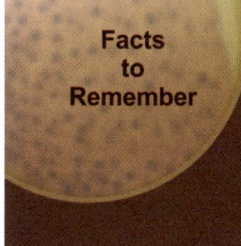

Facts to Remember

_____

_____

_____

KIDNEY

The kidney is covered by a connective tissue capsule. It is divided into an outer cortex which appears granular in a cut section, and an inner medulla.

Cortex of Kidney

_____

_____

_____

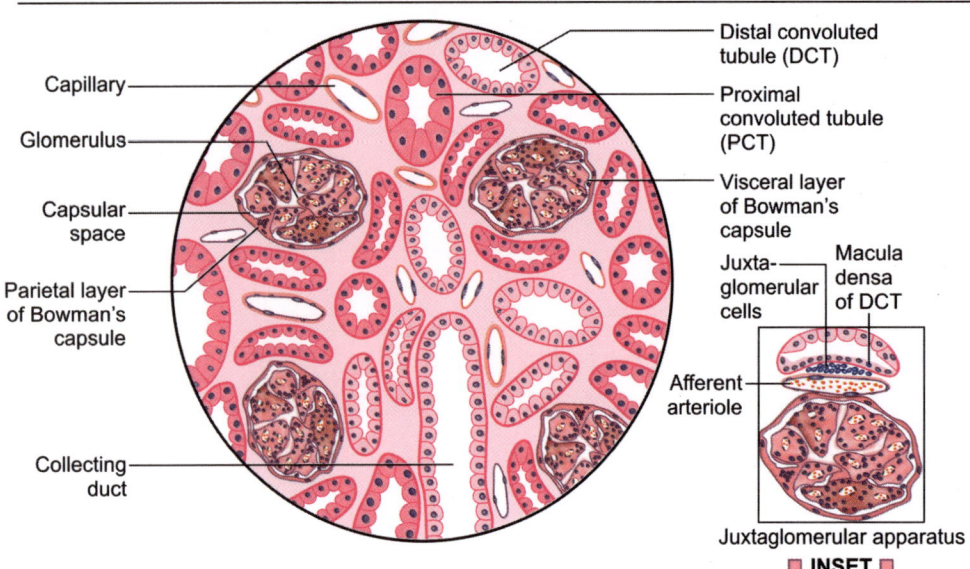

Cortex. Stain: Haematoxylin-eosin, 100X

Medulla of Kidney

_____

_____

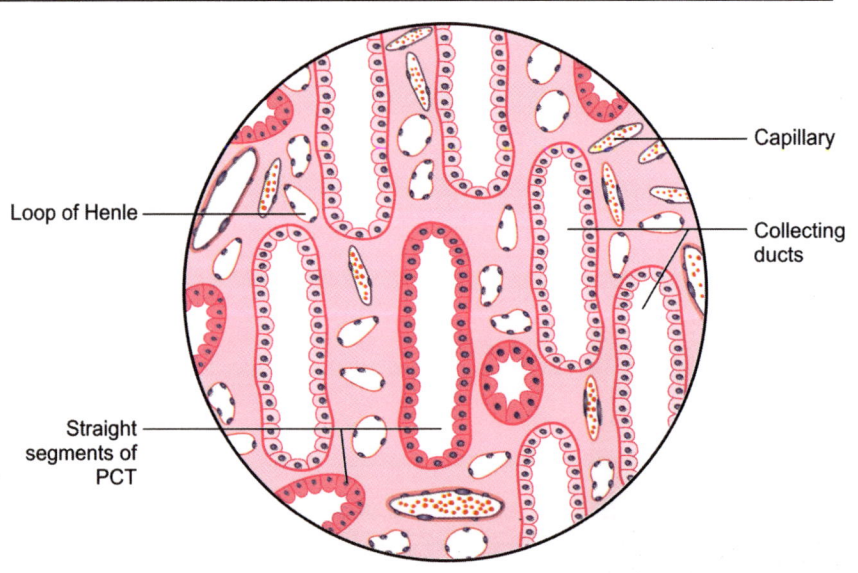

Medulla. Stain: Haematoxylin-eosin, 100X

Cortex of Kidney

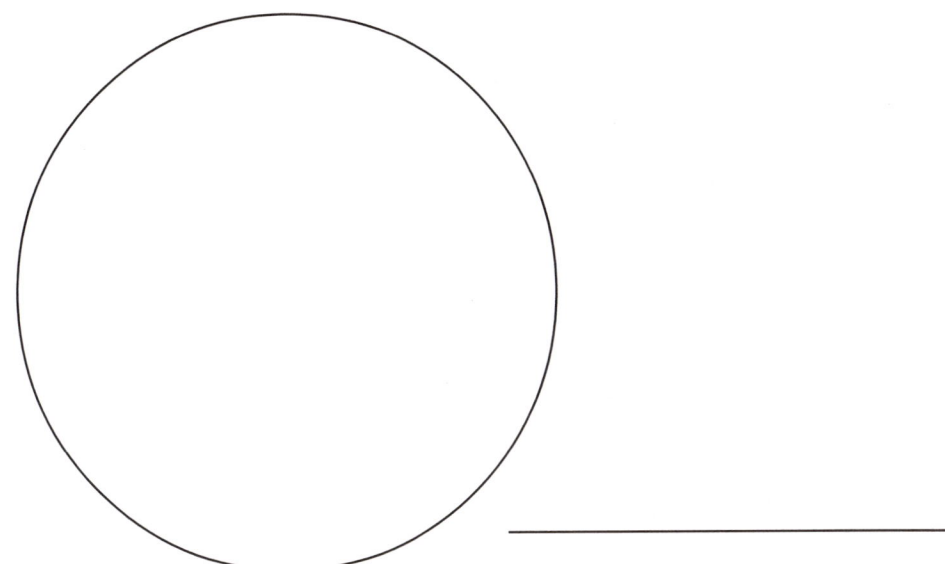

_____

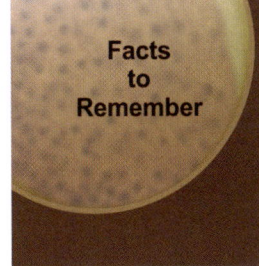

**Facts
to
Remember**

_____

_____

_____

Medulla of Kidney

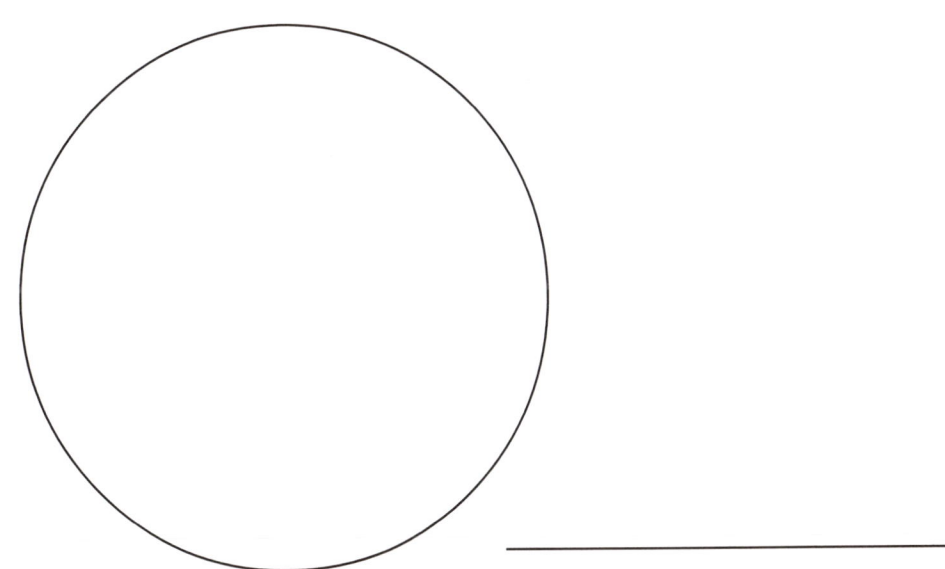

_____

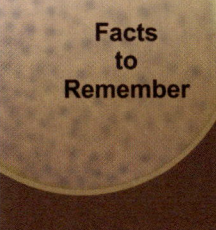

**Facts
to
Remember**

_____

_____

_____

URETER

The ureter is a muscular tube conveying urine formed by the kidneys to the urinary bladder where it is stored temporarily. The ureter consists of an inner mucous membrane, a middle well developed smooth muscle coat and outer tunica adventitia. The details are: _____

_____

_____

_____

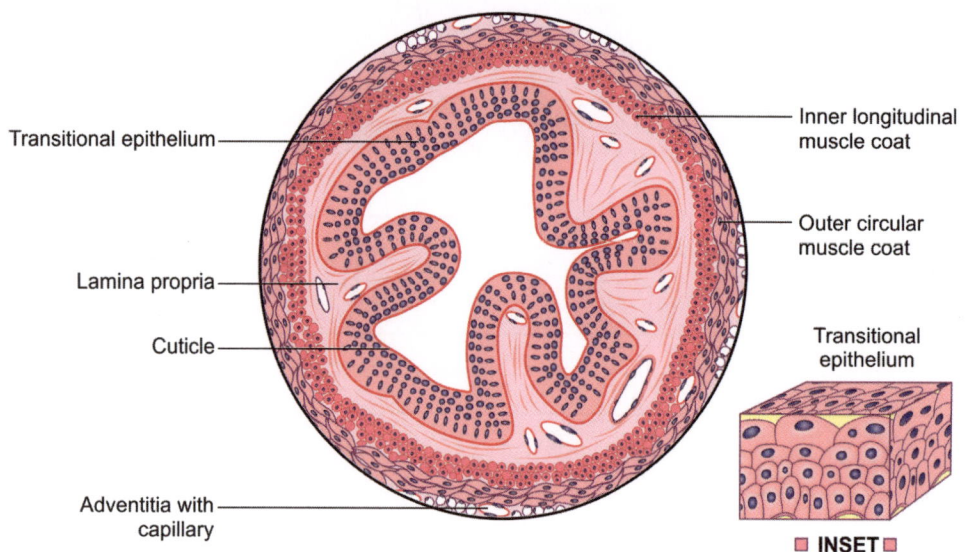

Transitional epithelium

Inner longitudinal muscle coat

Outer circular muscle coat

Transitional epithelium

Lamina propria

Cuticle

Adventitia with capillary

■ INSET ■

Ureter. Stain: Haematoxylin-eosin, 100X

URINARY BLADDER

The urinary bladder is a temporary waterproof storehouse of urine. Its wall is thicker and lumen is much bigger than that of ureter. It also comprises inner mucous coat, middle muscular coat and outer fibrous coat:

_____

_____

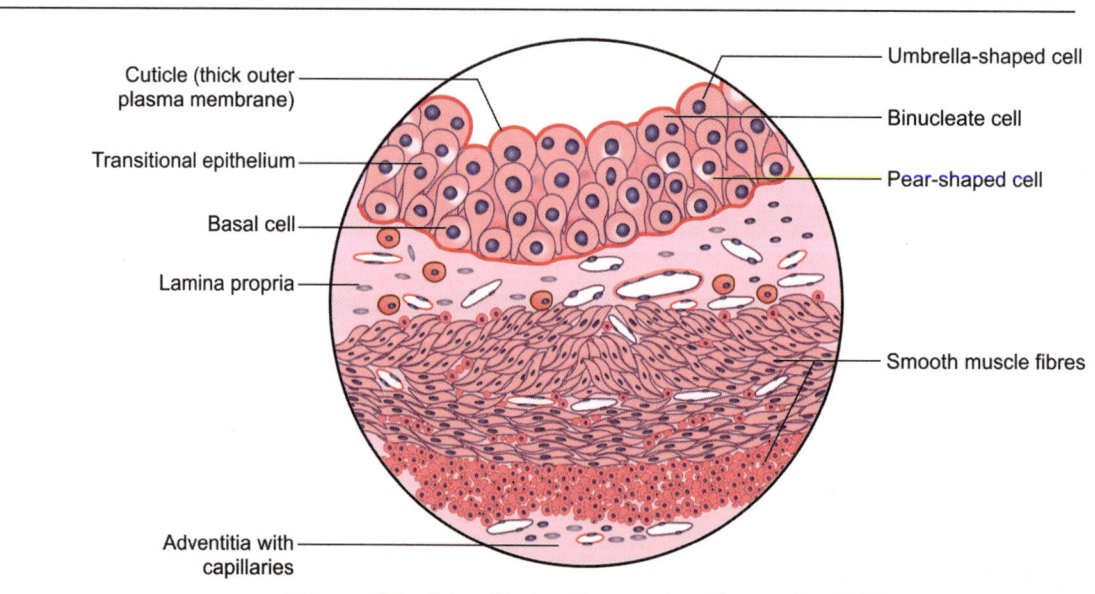

Cuticle (thick outer plasma membrane)

Umbrella-shaped cell

Binucleate cell

Transitional epithelium

Pear-shaped cell

Basal cell

Lamina propria

Smooth muscle fibres

Adventitia with capillaries

Urinary bladder. Stain: Haematoxylin-eosin, 400X

Ureter

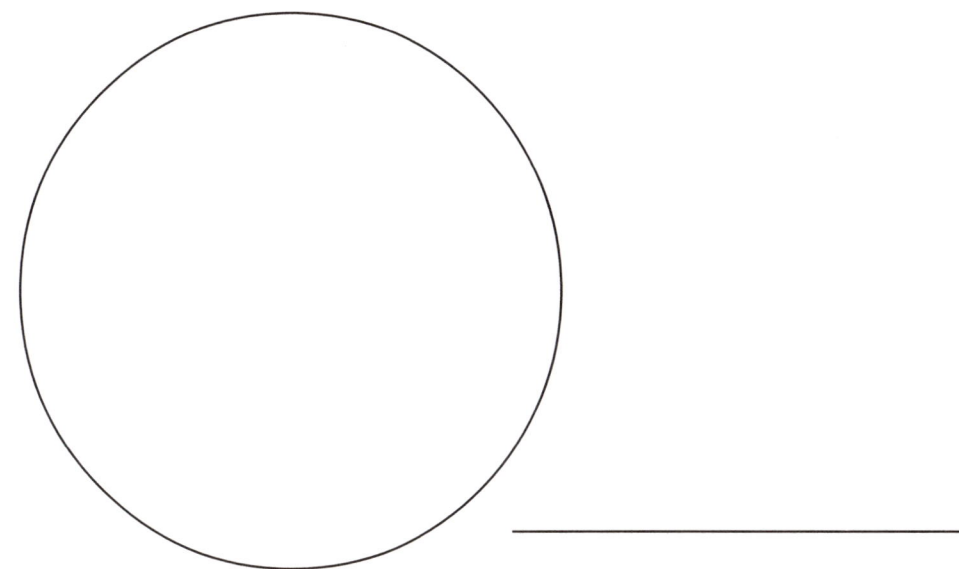

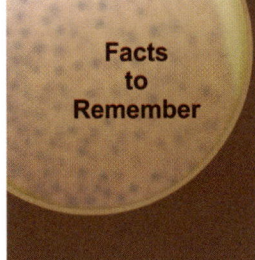

Facts to Remember

_____

_____

_____

Urinary Bladder

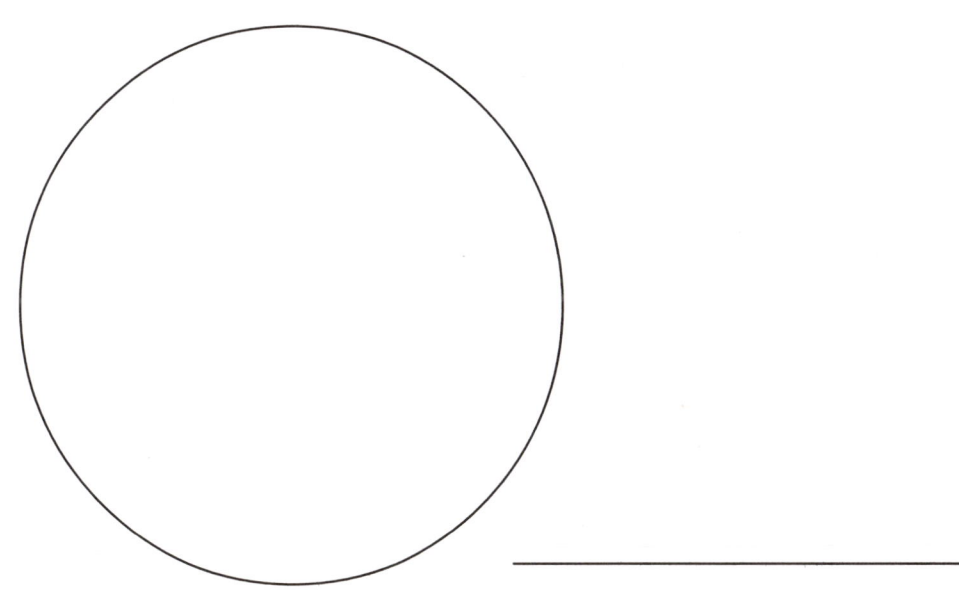

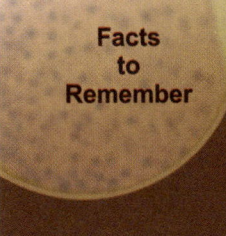

Facts to Remember

_____

_____

_____

ADDITIONAL FIGURES/NOTES

ADDITIONAL FIGURES/NOTES

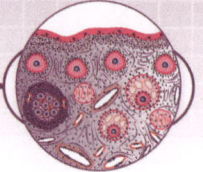

16. Male Reproductive System

TESTIS

The testis is divided by thin fibrous septa into various lobules. Each lobule contains one to four highly convoluted *seminiferous tubules*. The structure of testis is: _____

_____

_____

_____

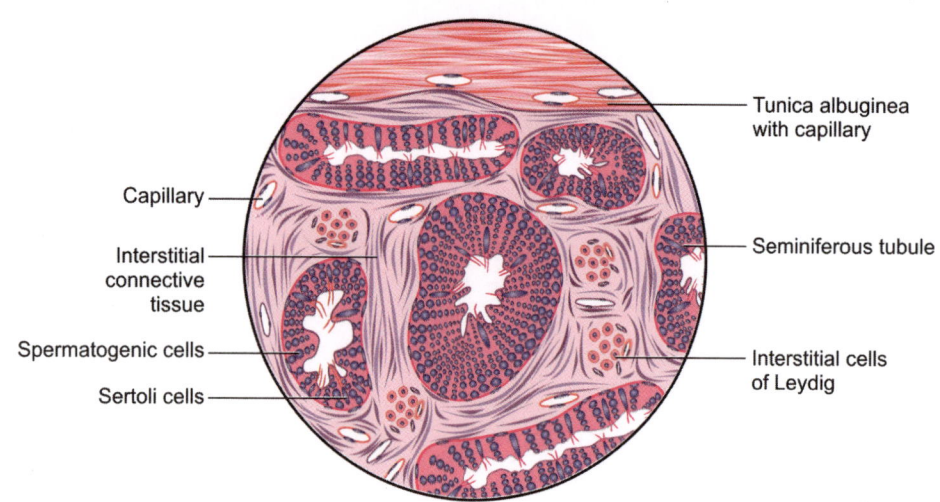

Testis. Stain: Haematoxylin-eosin, 100X

Seminiferous Tubule

The seminiferous tubule is lined by stratified epithelium 4–8 layers thick, composed of *supporting cells* and the *spermatogenic cells*. Various spermatogenic cells are: _____

_____

_____

_____

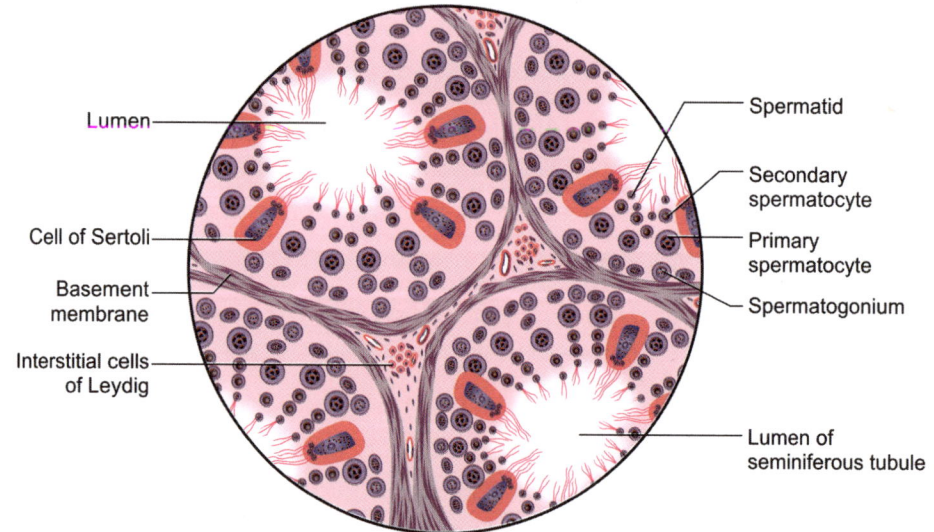

Seminiferous tubule. Stain: Haematoxylin-eosin, 400X

Testis

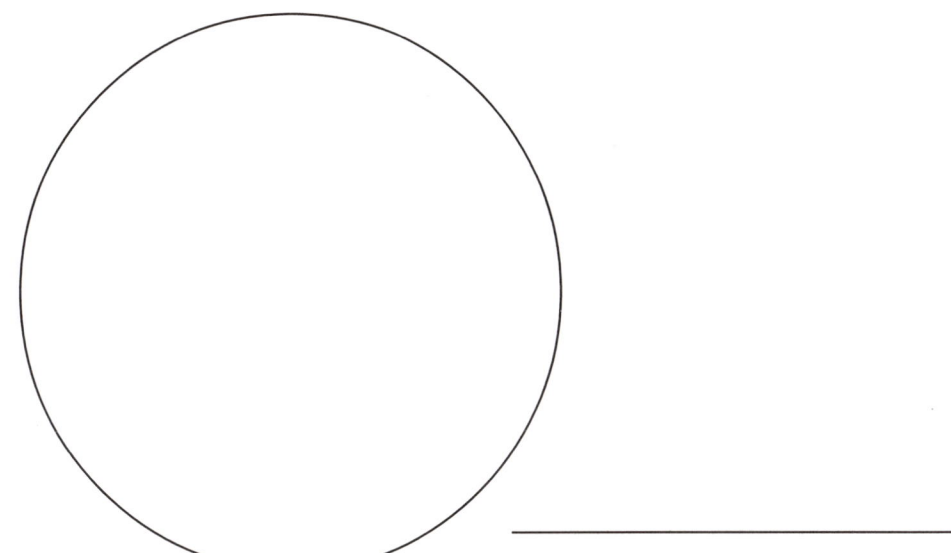

_____

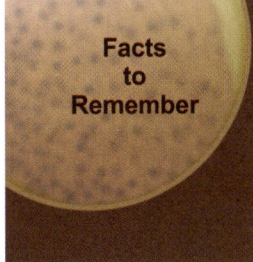

Facts to Remember

_____

_____

_____

Seminiferous Tubule

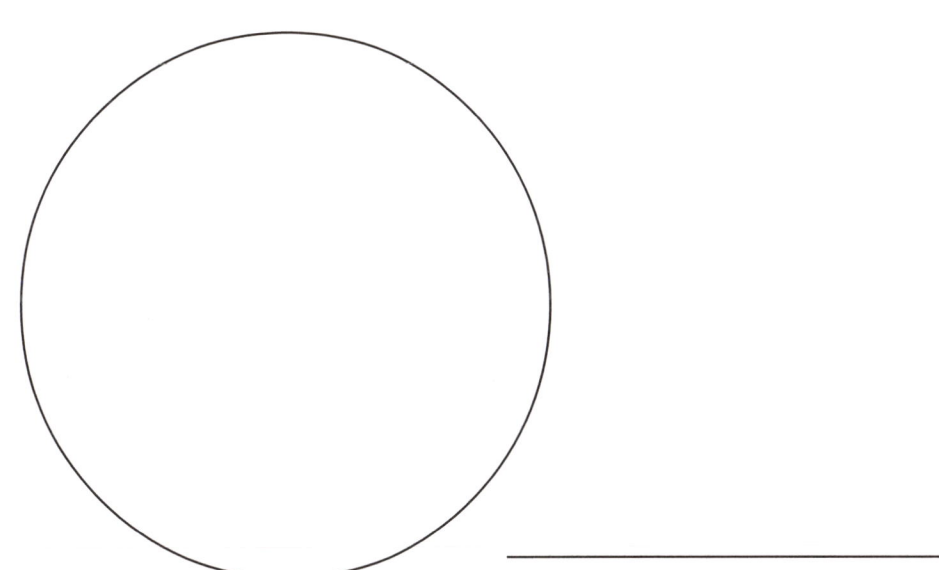

_____

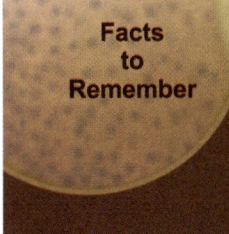

Facts to Remember

_____

_____

_____

EPIDIDYMIS

The structure of epididymis is: _____

_____

_____

_____

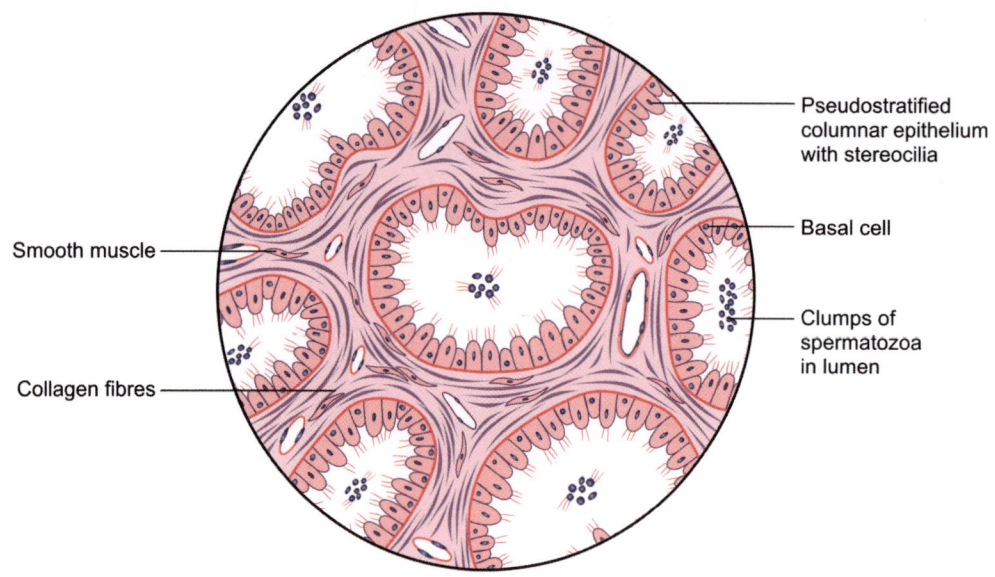

Pseudostratified columnar epithelium with stereocilia

Basal cell

Smooth muscle

Clumps of spermatozoa in lumen

Collagen fibres

Epididymis. Stain: Haematoxylin-eosin, 100X

DUCTUS DEFERENS

It is a thick muscular tube whose entire outer wall can be seen in single low power field of microscope. Its structure is:

_____

_____

_____

_____

Pseudostratified columnar epithelium

Inner longitudinal layer

Middle circular layer

Outer longitudinal layer

Lamina propria

Thick smooth muscle coat

Mucosal fold

Adventitia with fat cells

Ductus deferens. Stain: Haematoxylin-eosin, 100X

Epididymis

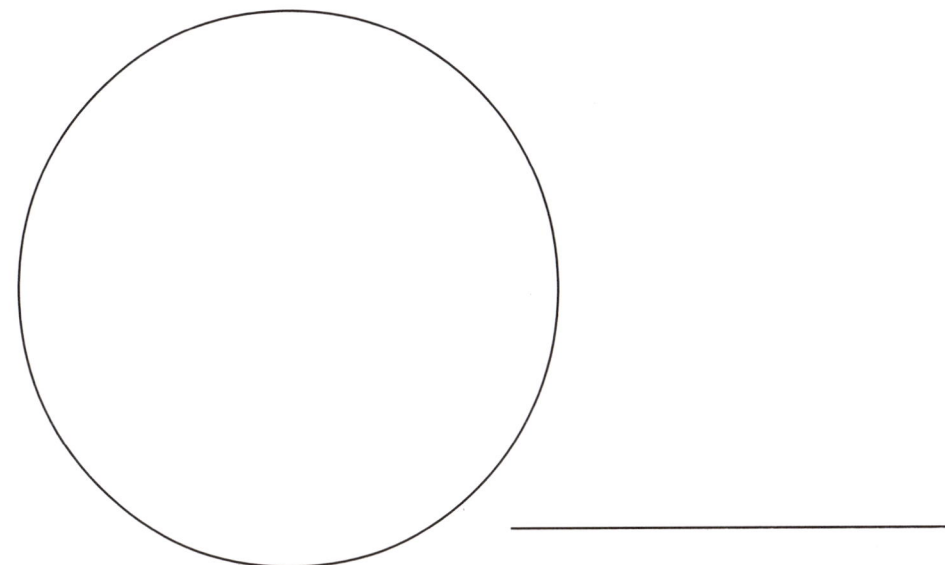

Ductus Deferens

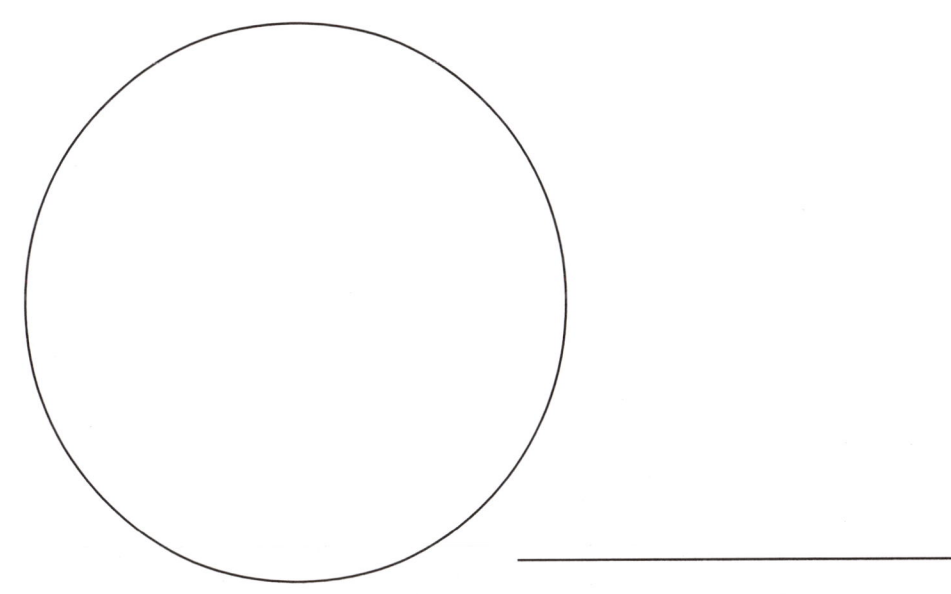

PROSTATE GLAND

Prostate gland is a fibromuscular glandular organ. Its structure is:

_____

_____

_____

_____

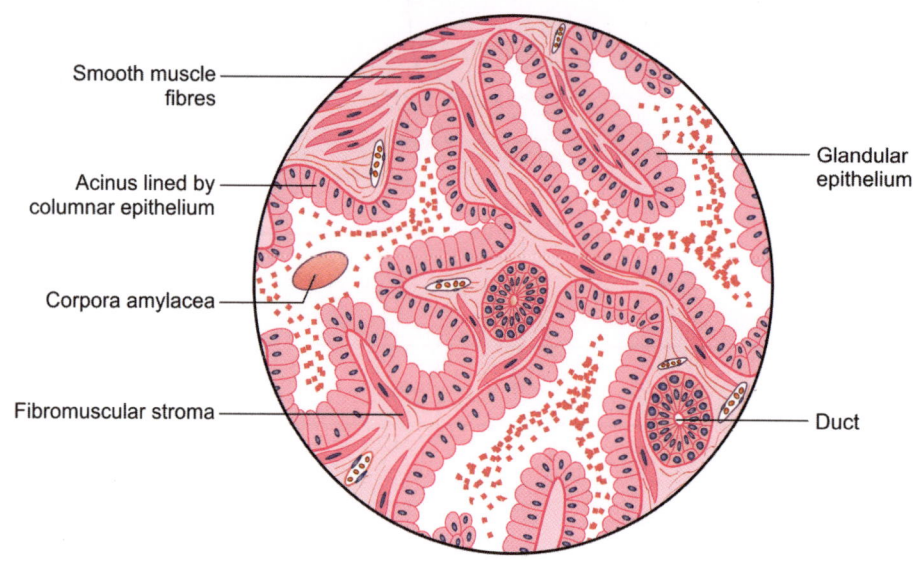

Prostate gland. Stain: Haematoxylin-eosin, 100X

SEMINAL VESICLE

Each seminal vesicle consists of highly tortuous tube about 15 cm in length. Its structure is:

_____

_____

_____

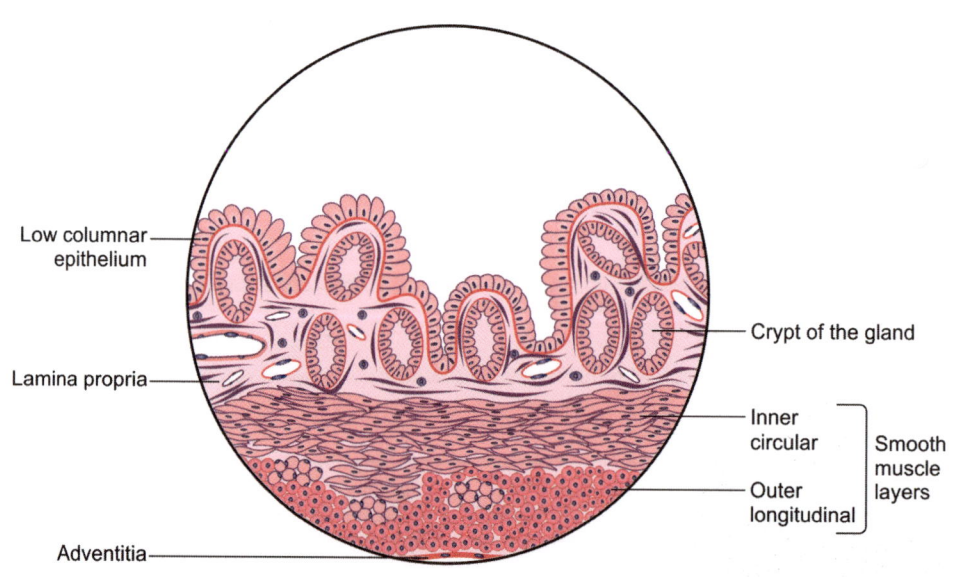

Seminal vesicle. Stain: Haematoxylin-eosin, 100X

Prostate Gland

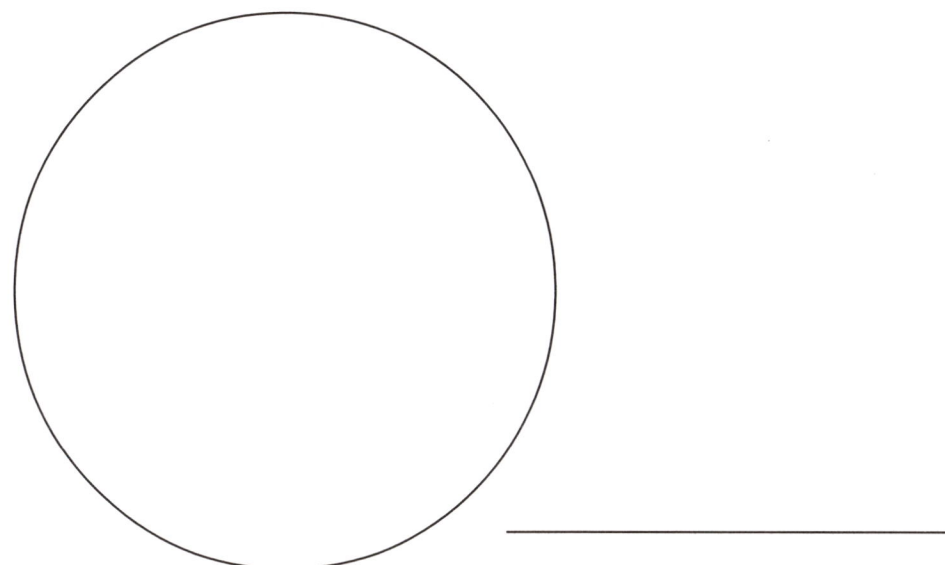

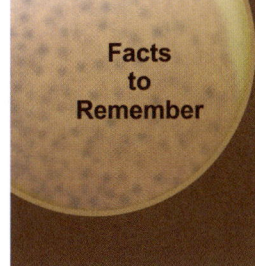

Facts
to
Remember

Seminal Vesicle

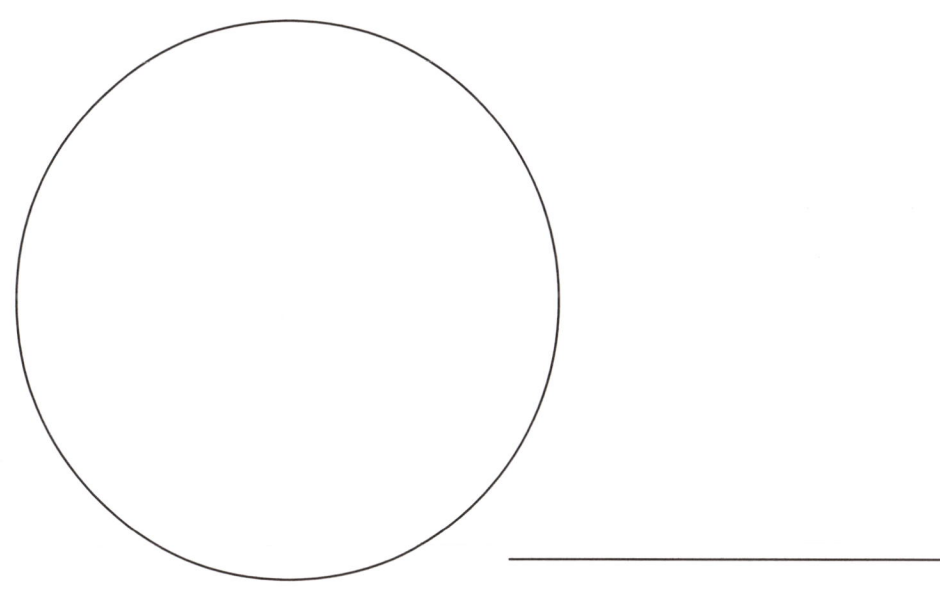

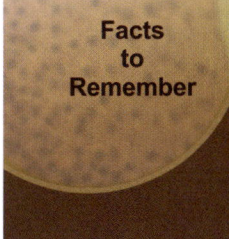

Facts
to
Remember

PENIS

Penis is the male copulatory organ. It subserves for the passage of both semen and urine. Penis consists of three cylindrical bodies of erectile or cavernous tissue. Two *corpora cavernosa* lying dorsally and a single *corpus spongiosum* situated on the ventral aspect.

_____

_____

_____

_____

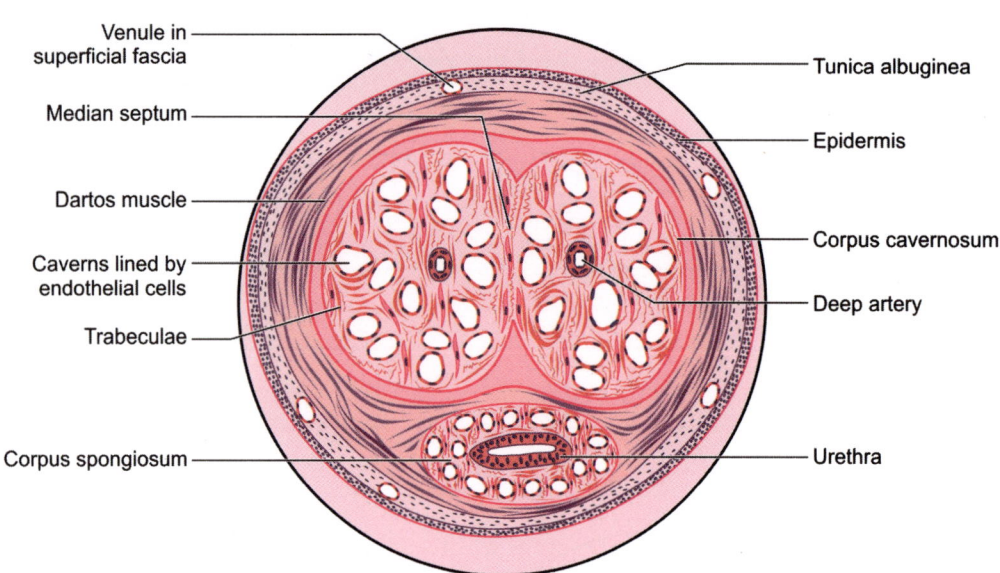

Penis. Stain: Haematoxylin-eosin, 20X

Penis

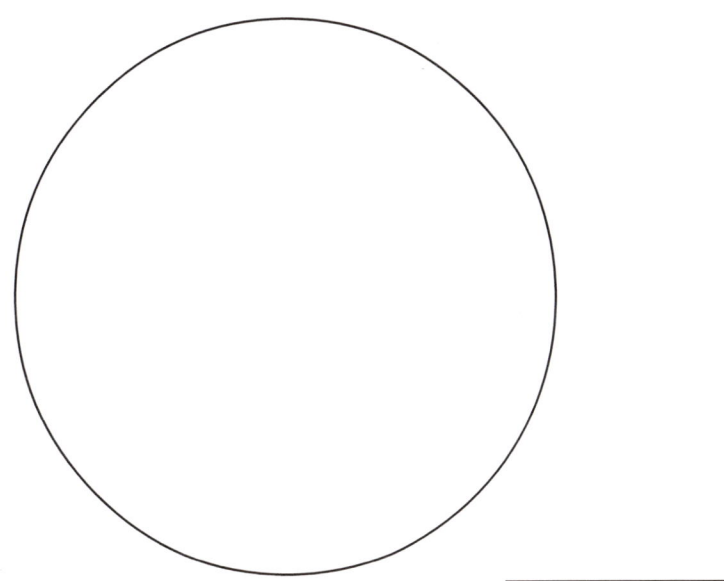

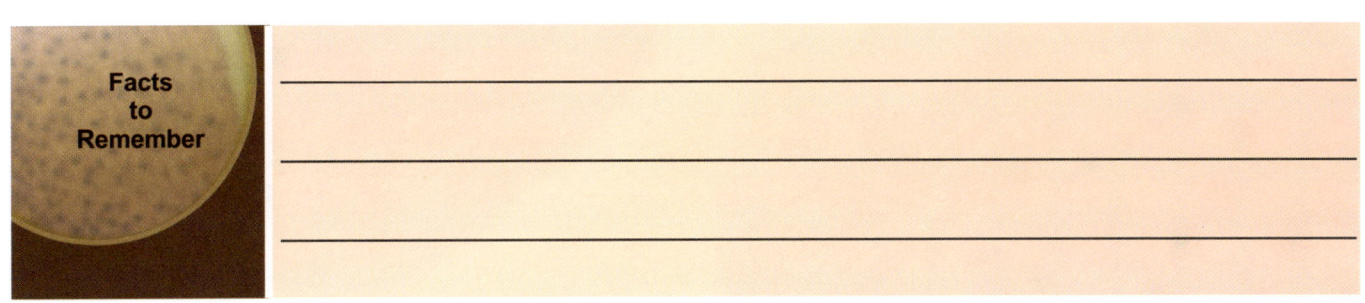

**Facts
to
Remember**

Notes

17. Female Reproductive System

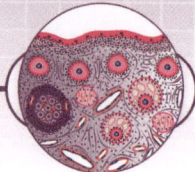

OVARY

The surface of the ovary is covered by *cuboidal epithelium*. The ovary consists of a thick peripheral or outer cortex which surrounds the inner *medulla*.

Cortex: _____

_____

_____

Ovary. Stain: Haematoxylin-eosin, 100X

Graafian Follicle

_____

_____

_____

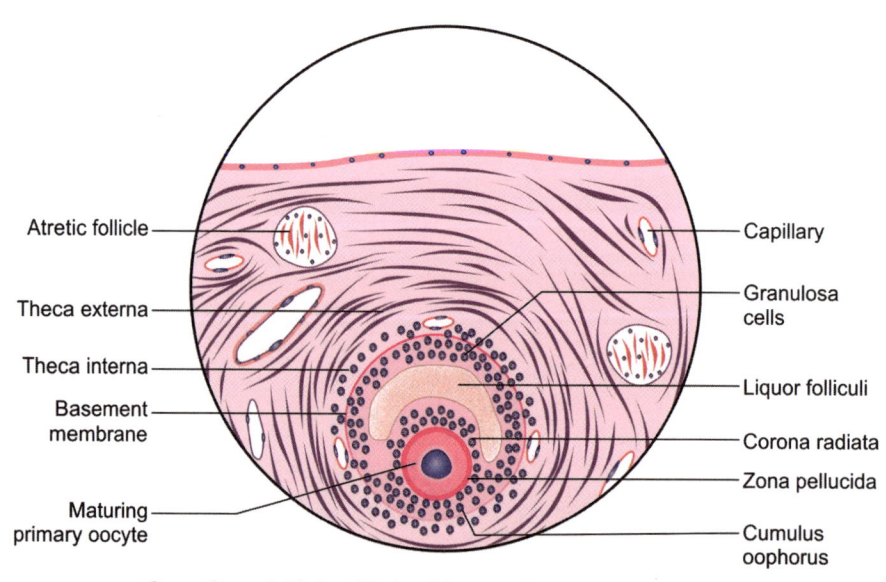

Graafian follicle. Stain: Haematoxylin-eosin, 400X

Ovary

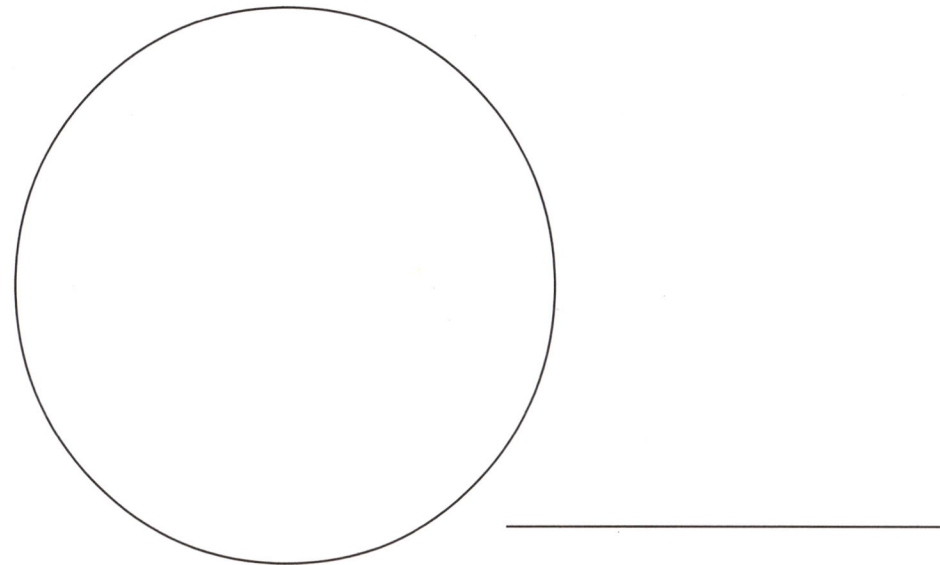

_____

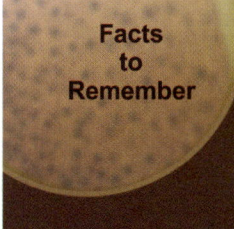

Facts to Remember

_____

_____

_____

Graafian Follicle

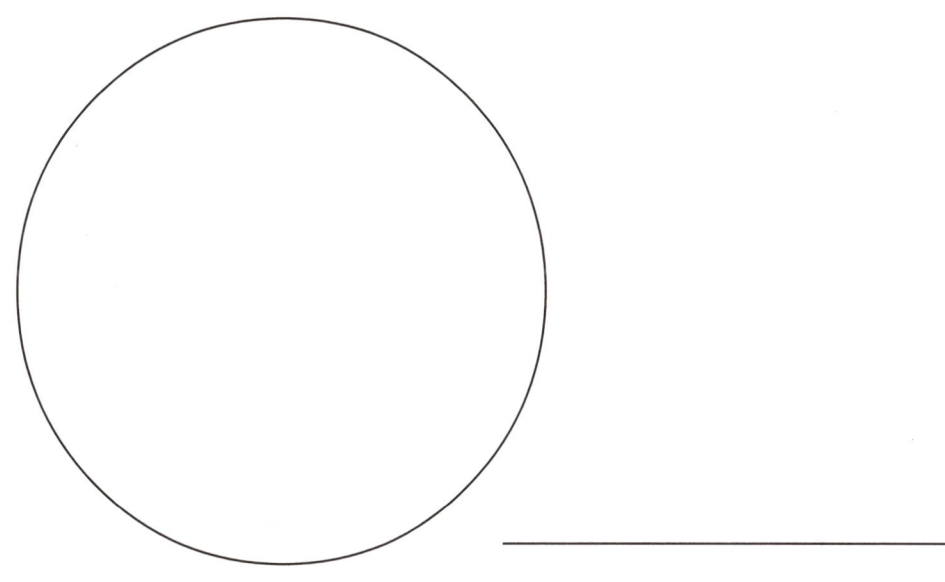

_____

Facts to Remember

_____

_____

_____

FALLOPIAN TUBE OR OVIDUCT

Fallopian tube is the part of female reproductive tract that receives the secondary oocyte, provides the appropriate environment for its fertilisation and transports it to the uterus. Its parts from medial to lateral are *intramural part*, *isthmus*, *ampulla* infundibulum with *fimbriae*. It comprises following layers: _____

_____

_____

_____

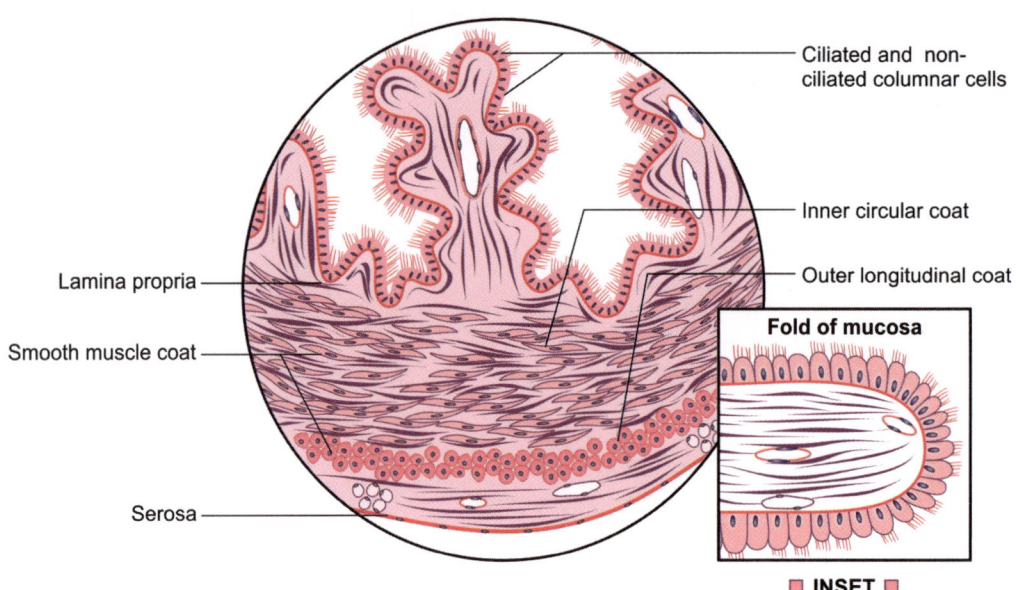

Ciliated and non-ciliated columnar cells

Inner circular coat

Outer longitudinal coat

Fold of mucosa

Lamina propria

Smooth muscle coat

Serosa

◼ **INSET** ◼

Fallopian tube. Stain: Haematoxylin-eosin, 100X

UTERUS

Wall of the uterus consists of *endometrium*, the inner most lining; *myometrium*, the muscle coat and outer most the *peritoneum*. Beginning at puberty till menopause, the uterine endometrium undergoes monthly cyclic changes in structure. The cyclic activity of the non-pregnant uterus may be divided into three phases of the endometrium.

Uterus—Follicular or Proliferative Phase

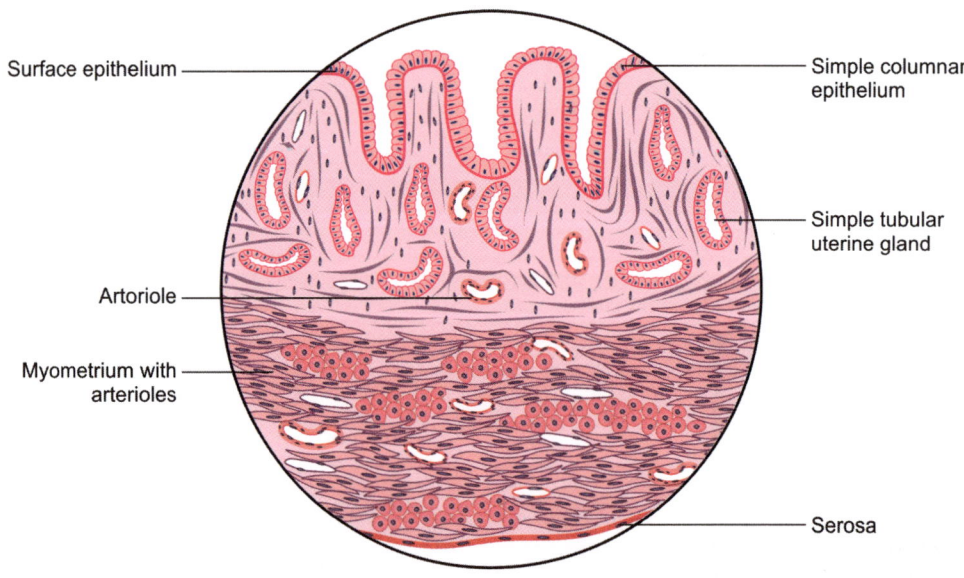

Surface epithelium

Simple columnar epithelium

Simple tubular uterine gland

Artoriole

Myometrium with arterioles

Serosa

Proliferative phase. Stain: Haematoxylin-eosin, 100X

Fallopian Tube or Oviduct

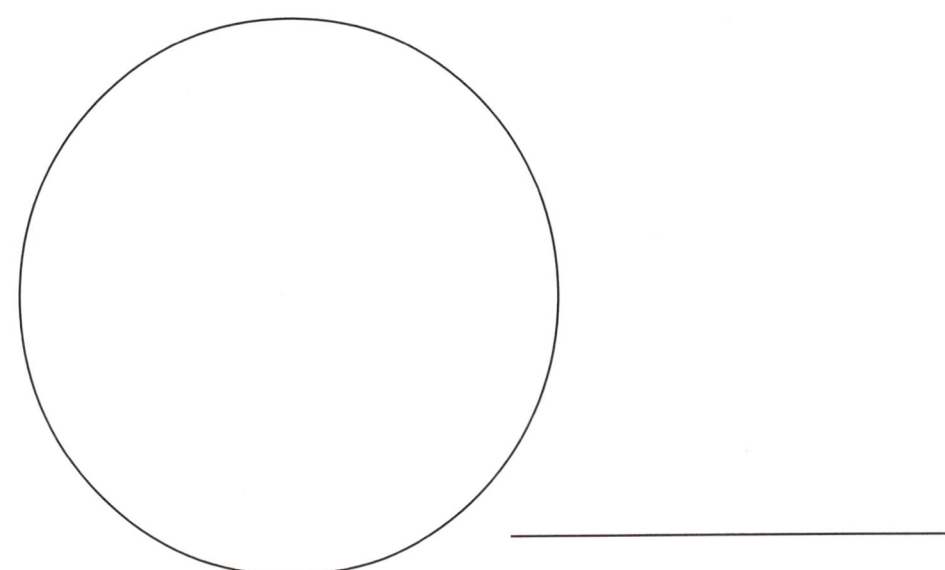

_____

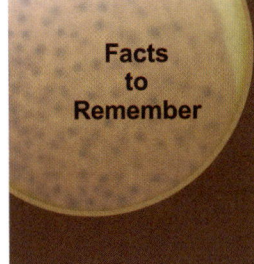

Facts to Remember

_____

_____

_____

Uterus—Follicular or Proliferative Phase

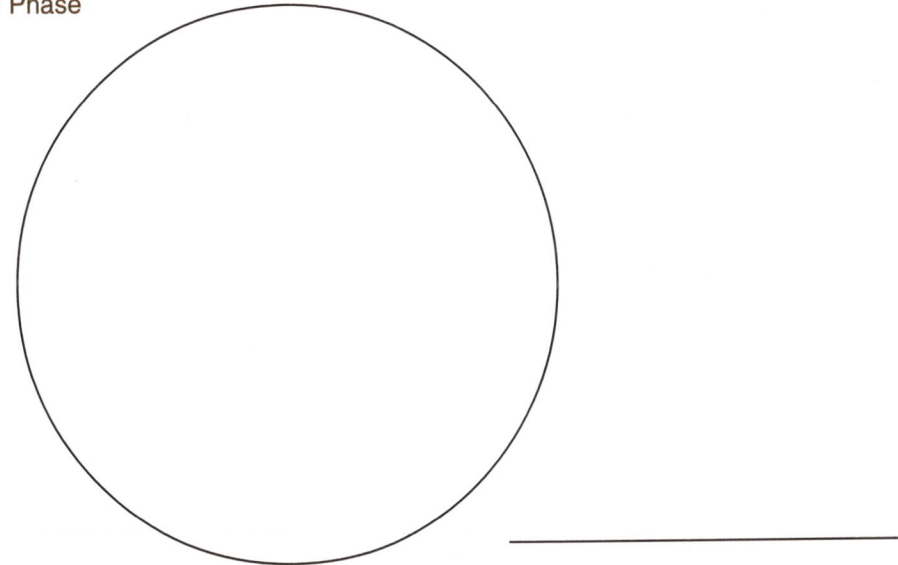

_____

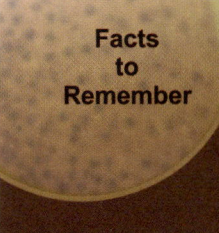

Facts to Remember

_____

_____

_____

Uterus—Progestational Phase

_____

_____

_____

_____

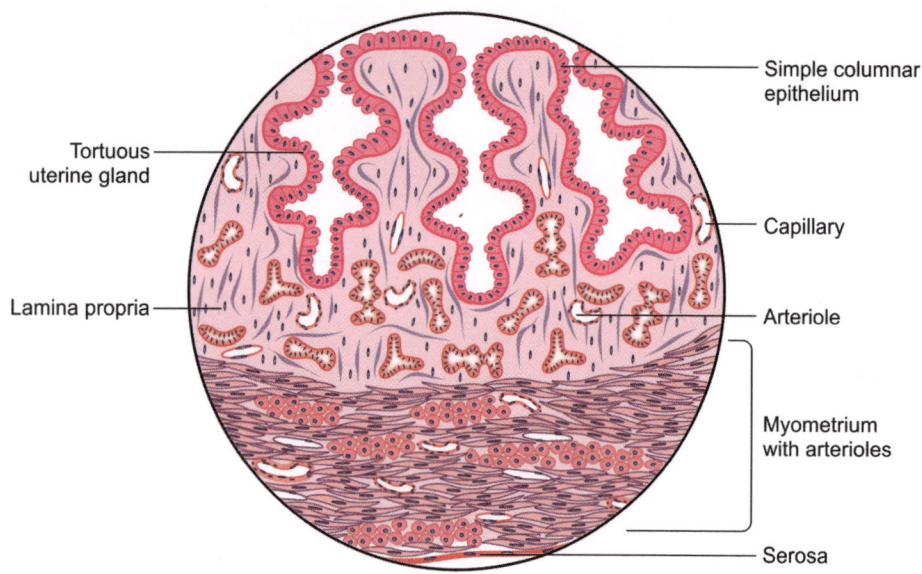

Progestational phase. Stain: Haematoxylin-eosin, 100X

Uterus—Menstrual Phase

_____

_____

_____

_____

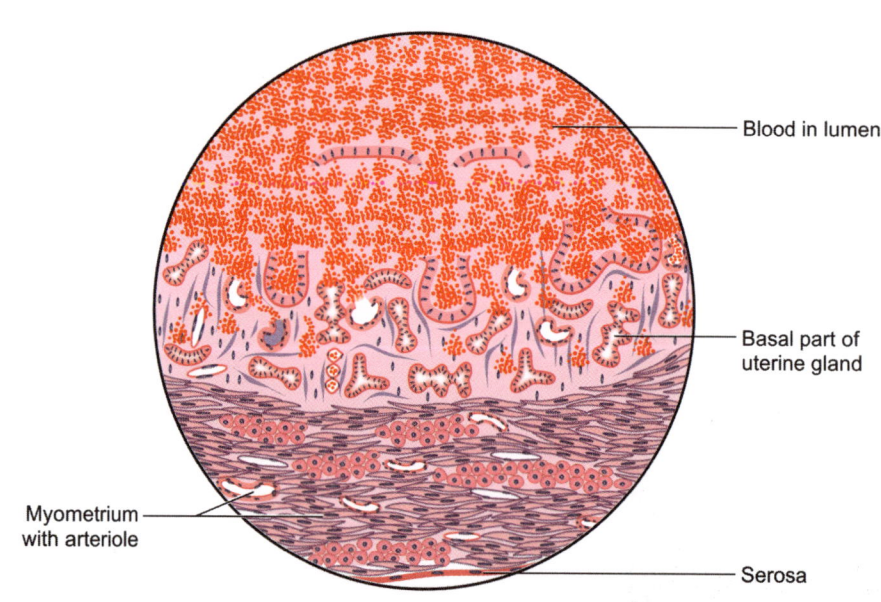

Menstrual phase. Stain: Haematoxylin-eosin, 100X

Uterus—Progestational Phase

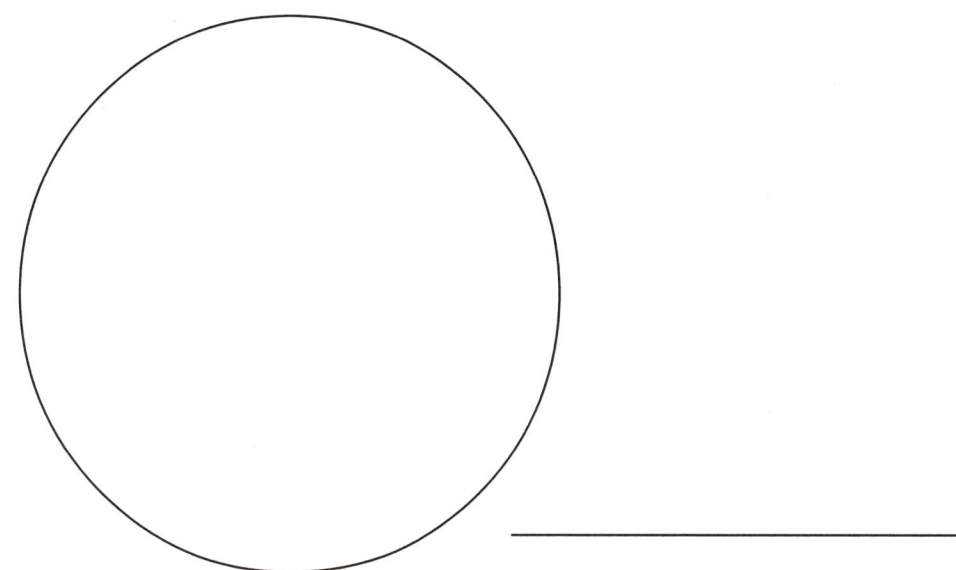

_____

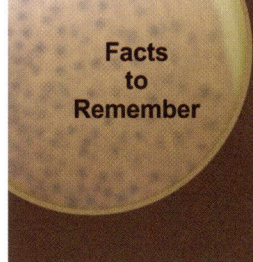

**Facts
to
Remember**

_____

_____

_____

Uterus—Menstrual Phase

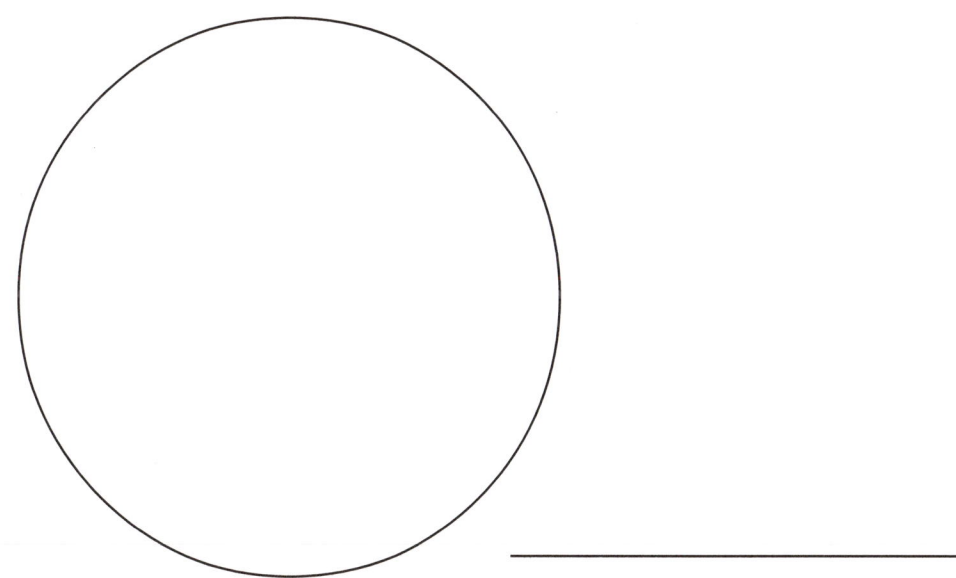

_____

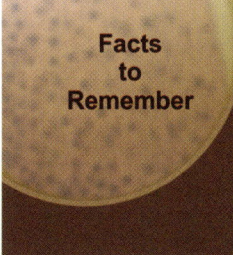

**Facts
to
Remember**

_____

_____

_____

Cervix

_____

_____

_____

_____

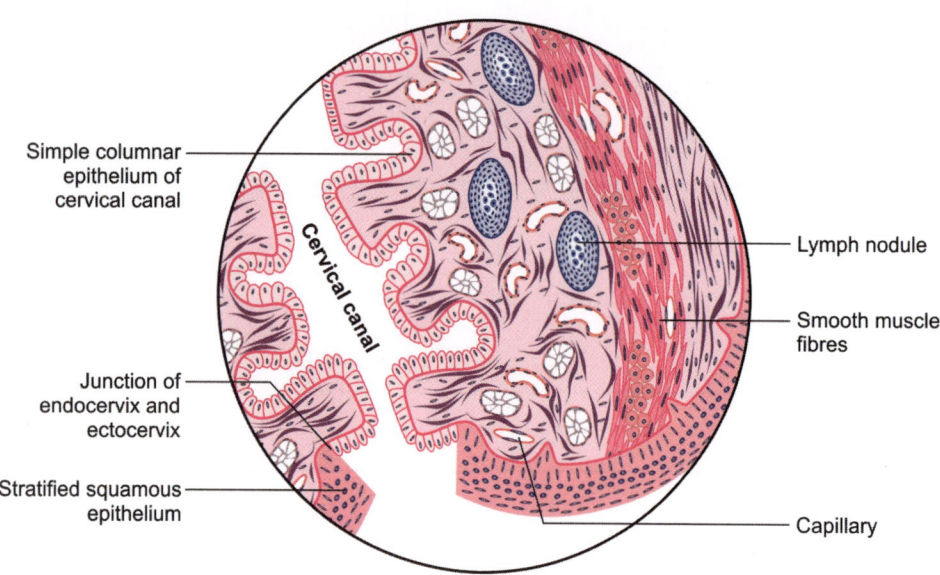

Simple columnar epithelium of cervical canal

Cervical canal

Junction of endocervix and ectocervix

Stratified squamous epithelium

Lymph nodule

Smooth muscle fibres

Capillary

Cervix. Stain: Haematoxylin-eosin, 100X

VAGINA

_____

_____

_____

_____

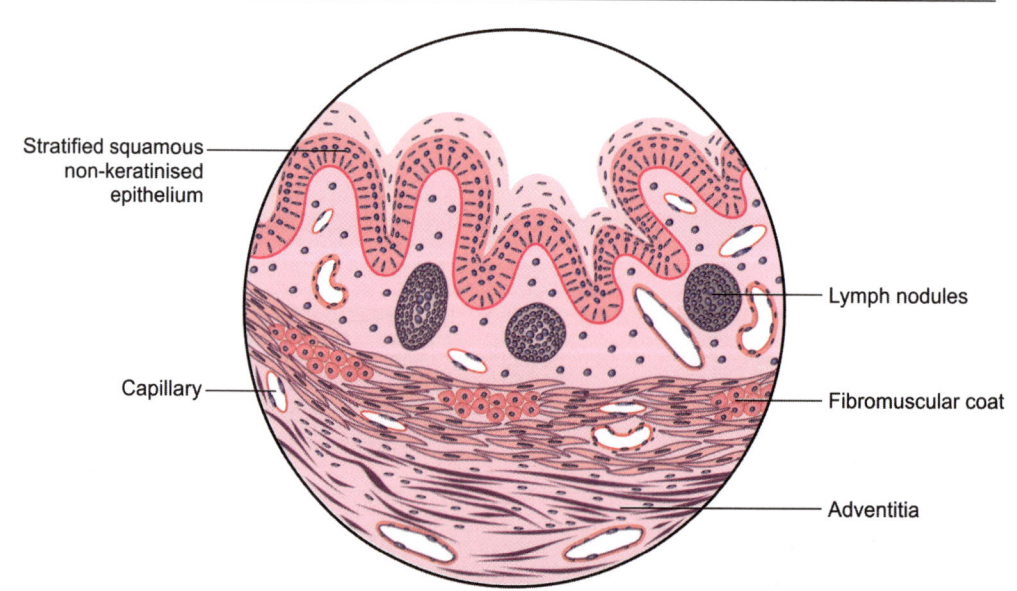

Stratified squamous non-keratinised epithelium

Capillary

Lymph nodules

Fibromuscular coat

Adventitia

Vagina. Stain: Haematoxylin-eosin, 100X

Cervix

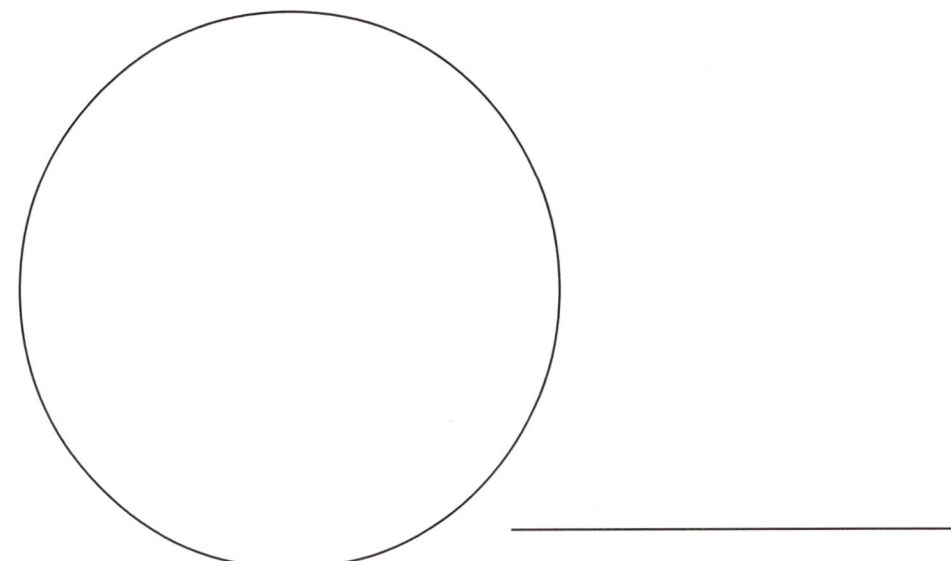

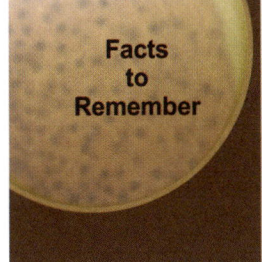

Facts to Remember

Vagina

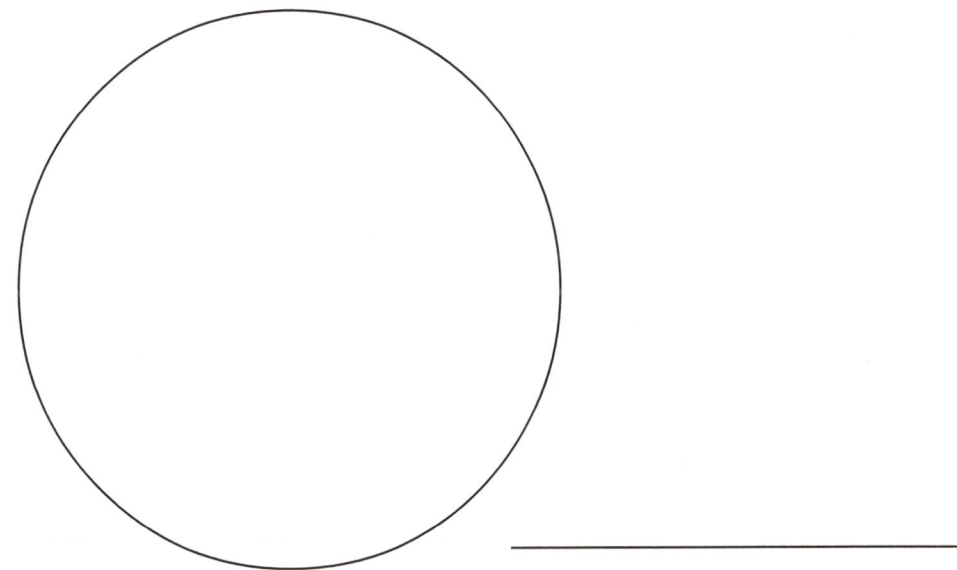

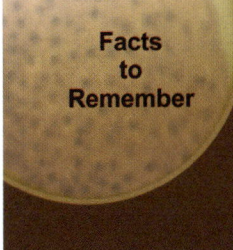

Facts to Remember

MAMMARY GLANDS

Mammary gland consists of 15–20 lobes with the same number of ducts. Each lobe is made up of many lobules containing acini. Histologically only lobules are discernible in the gland.

Resting Phase in Non-pregnant Adult Female

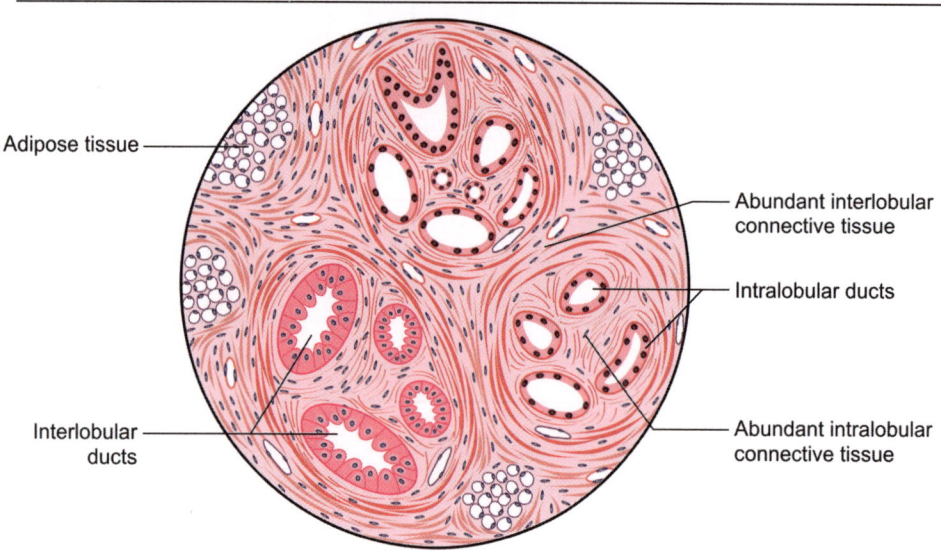

Resting phase. Stain: Haematoxylin-eosin, 100X

Lactating Phase

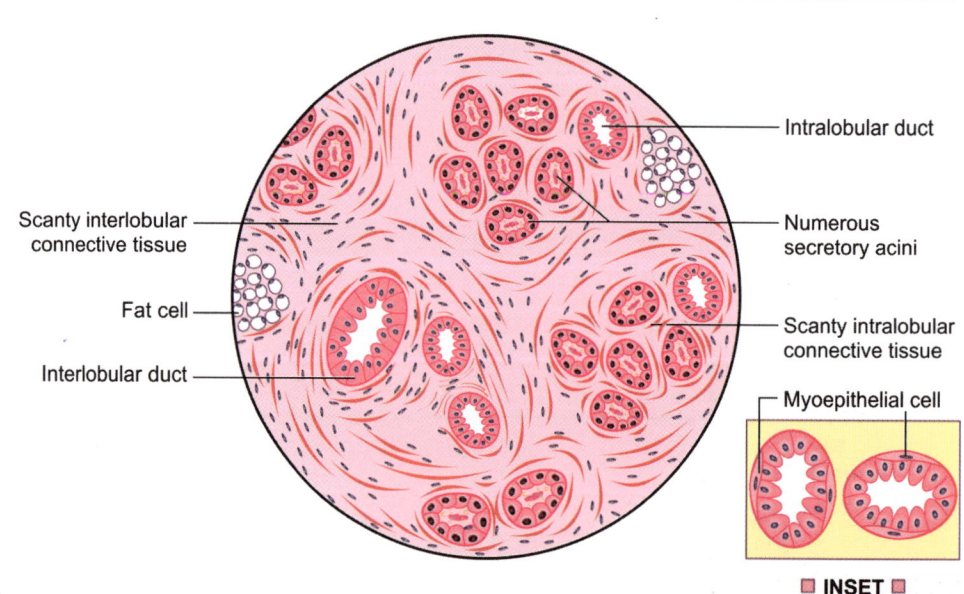

Lactating phase. Stain: Haematoxylin-eosin, 100X

Resting Phase

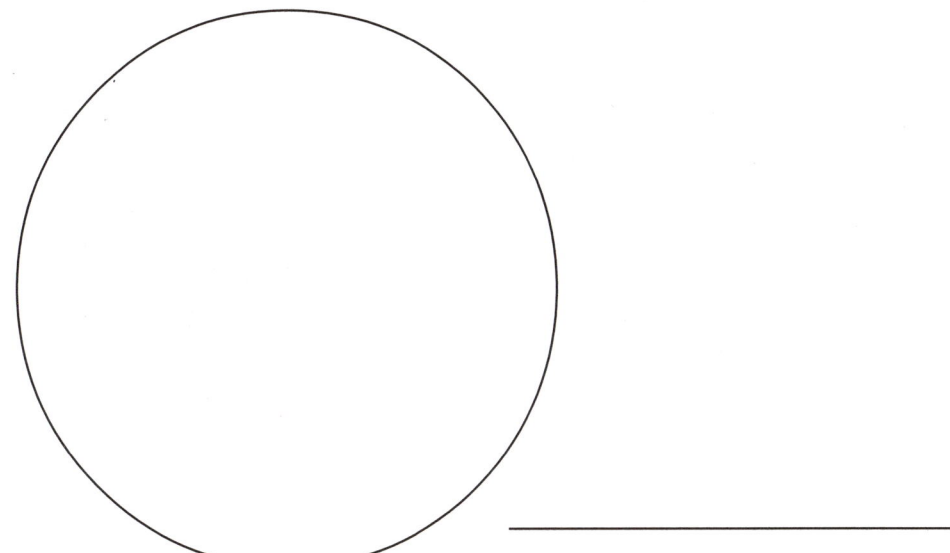

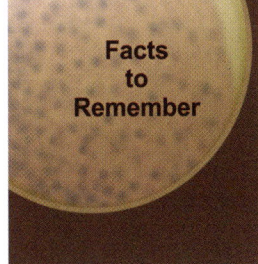

Facts
to
Remember

Lactating Phase

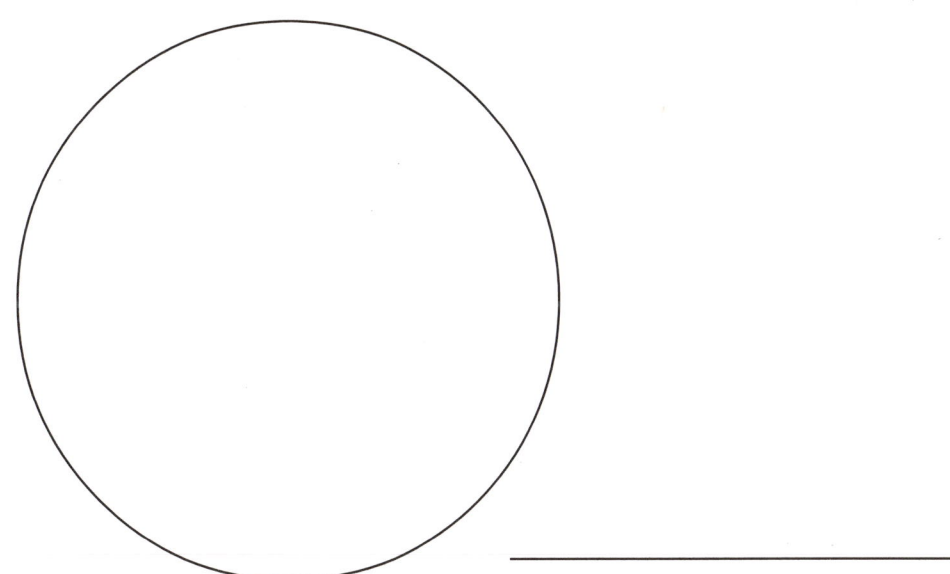

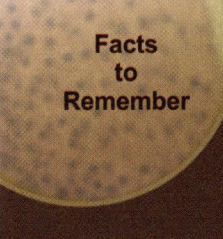

Facts
to
Remember

PLACENTA

Placenta—5th Month of Pregnancy

Placenta is fully formed and functional by three months of pregnancy. The villi of a foetus at five months of pregnancy shows cut sections of several chorionic villi. The structure of villus is:

_____

_____

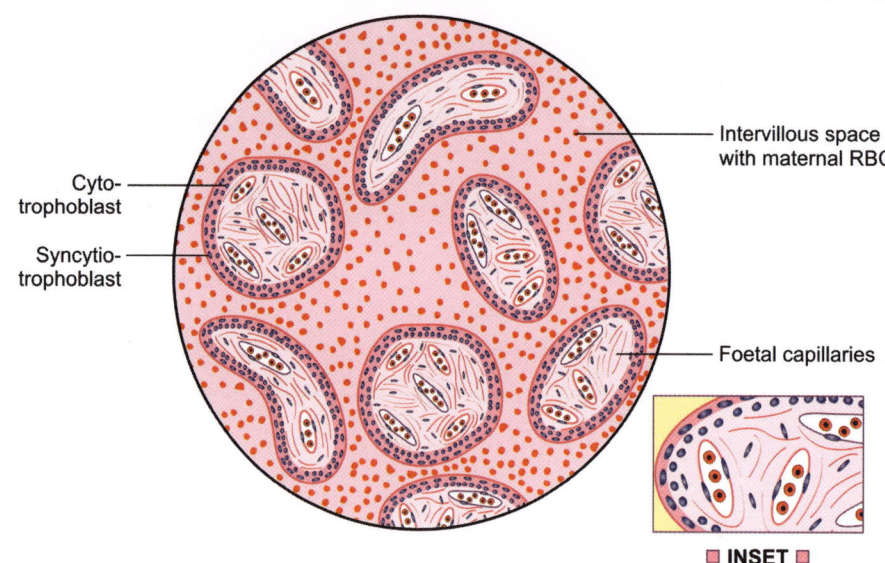

Placenta at 5 months. Stain: Haematoxylin-eosin, 100X

Placenta at Full Term

The chorionic villi of the placenta at full term show the chorionic epithelium only as syncytial trophoblast. Cytotrophoblast starts disappearing after five months of pregnancy and the foetal capillaries increase in number.

Placental Barrier

_____

_____

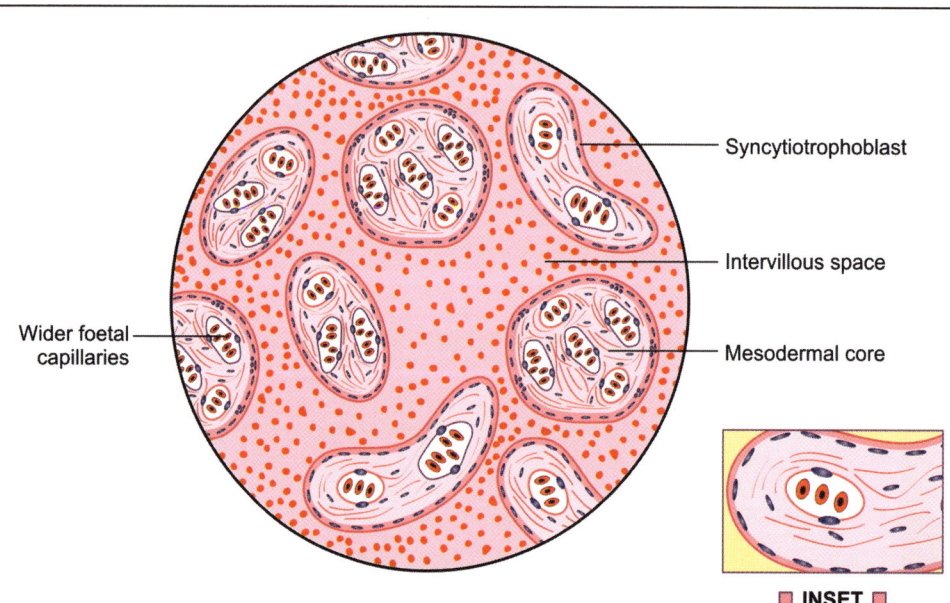

Placenta at full term. Stain: Haematoxylin-eosin, 100X

Placenta—5th Month of Pregnancy

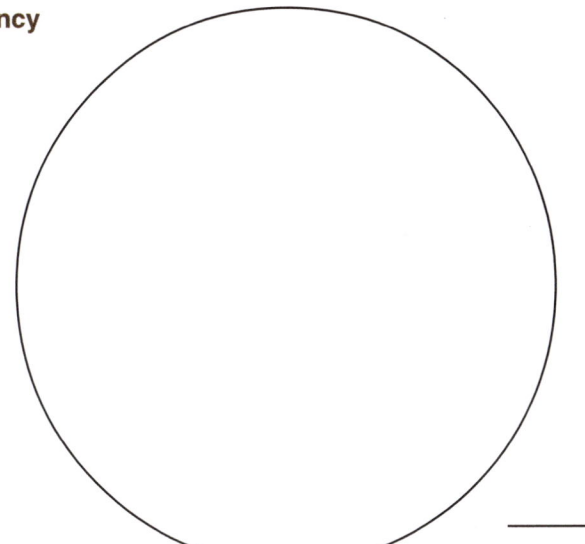

_____

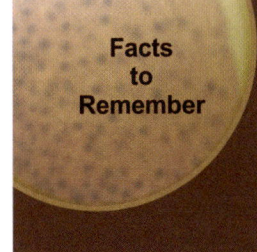

**Facts
to
Remember**

_____

_____

_____

Placenta at Full Term

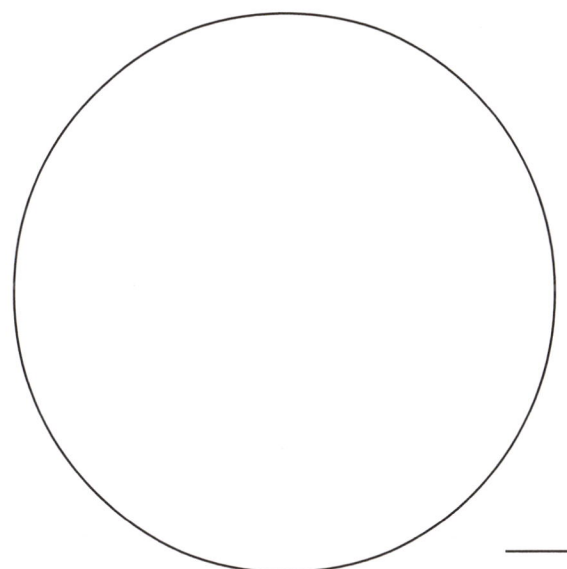

_____

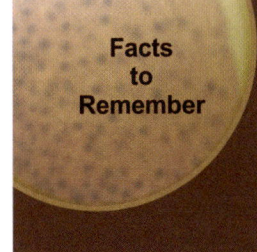

**Facts
to
Remember**

_____

_____

_____

UMBILICAL CORD

The umbilical cord approximately 50 cm long at full term connects the placenta to the foetus. It is the **lifeline of foetus**. Structures within the umbilical cord are: _____

_____

_____

_____

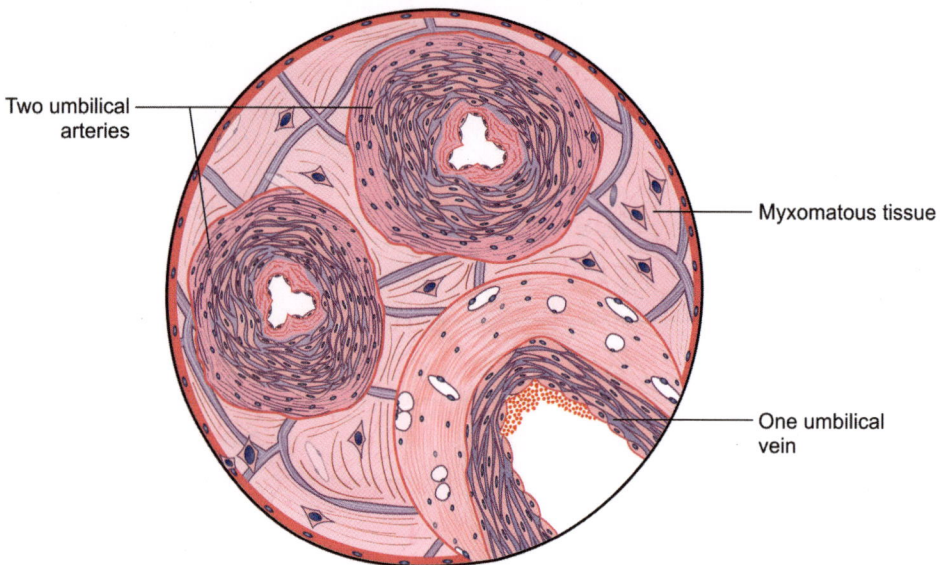

Two umbilical arteries

Myxomatous tissue

One umbilical vein

Umbilical cord. Stain: Haematoxylin-eosin, 100X

Notes

Umbilical Cord

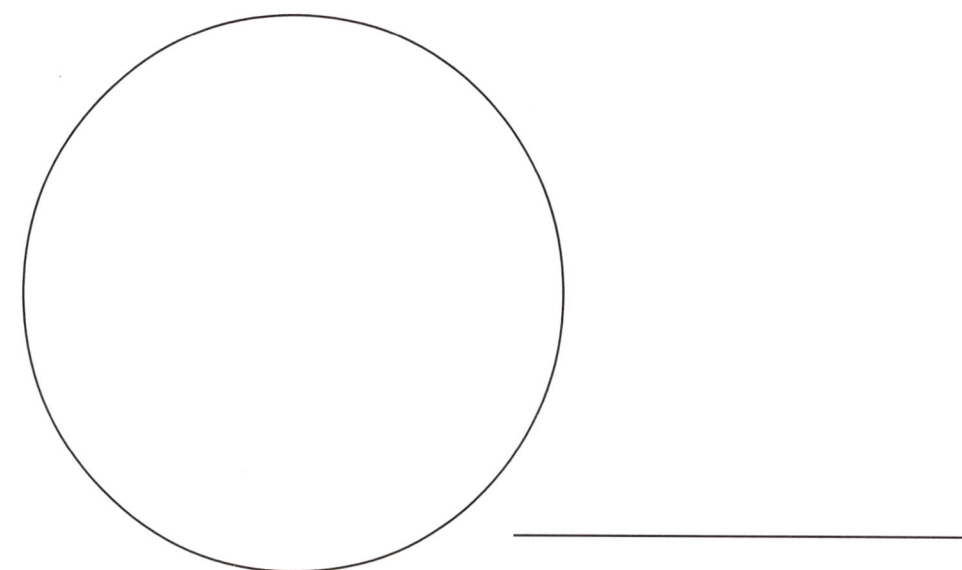

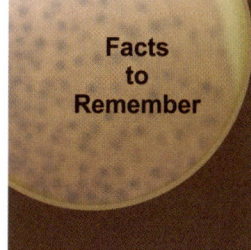

**Facts
to
Remember**

18. Endocrine Glands

HYPOPHYSIS CEREBRI

The hypophysis has two major divisions; the *neurohypophysis/posterior lobe* and *adenohypophysis* comprising the *pars distalis* or anterior lobe, *pars intermedia* and *pars tuberalis*.

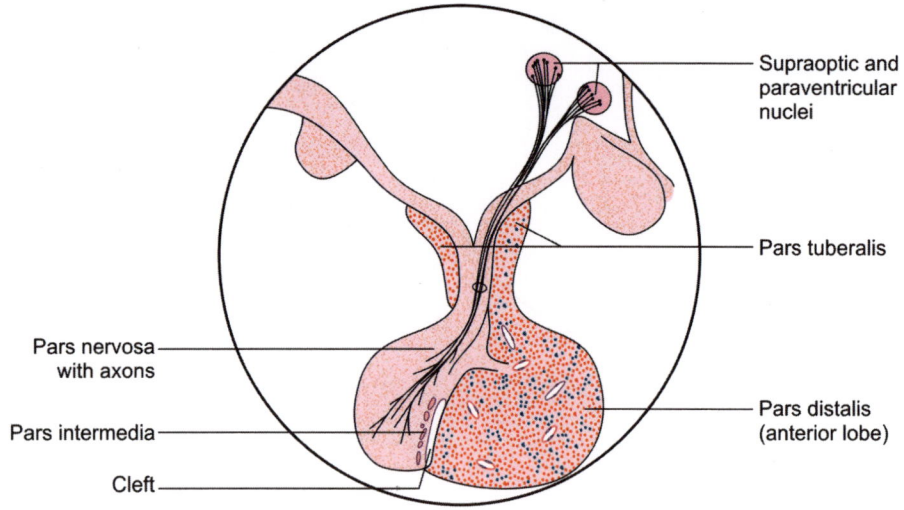

Supraoptic and paraventricular nuclei

Pars tuberalis

Pars nervosa with axons

Pars intermedia

Cleft

Pars distalis (anterior lobe)

Hypophysis cerebri. Stain: Haematoxylin-eosin, 20X

Pars Distalis

_____
_____
_____

Pars Intermedia

_____
_____

Pars Nervosa

_____
_____

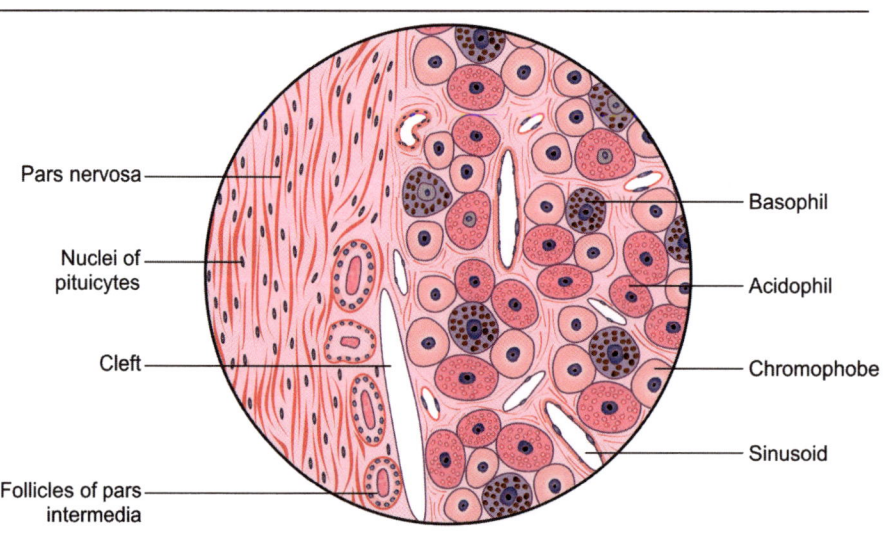

Pars nervosa

Nuclei of pituicytes

Cleft

Follicles of pars intermedia

Basophil

Acidophil

Chromophobe

Sinusoid

Hypophysis cerebri. Stain: Haematoxylin-eosin, 400X

Pars Distalis and Pars Intermedia

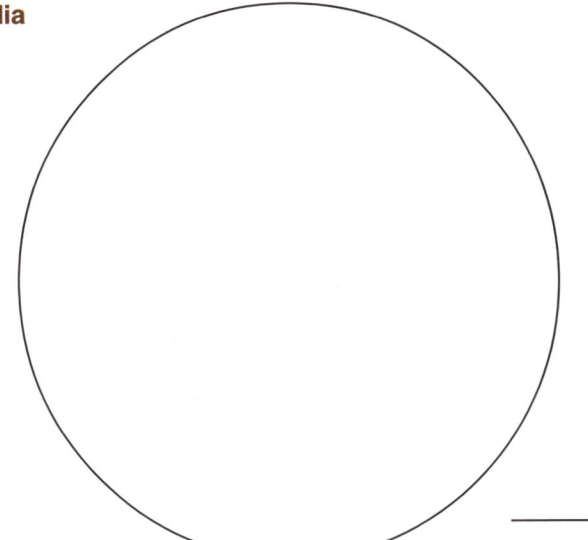

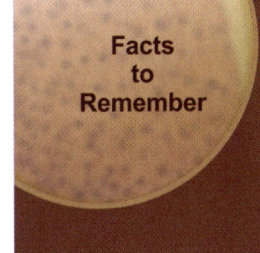

**Facts
to
Remember**

Pars Nervosa

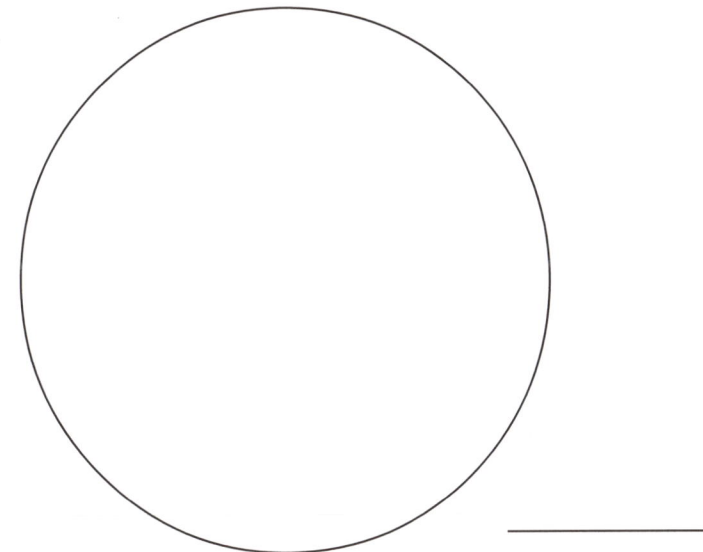

**Facts
to
Remember**

THYROID GLAND

Thyroid gland is responsible for maintaining the *basal metabolic rate* of the body. The gland is divided is lobes and lobules. The structural and functional unit of thyroid gland is a *follicle*.

_____

_____

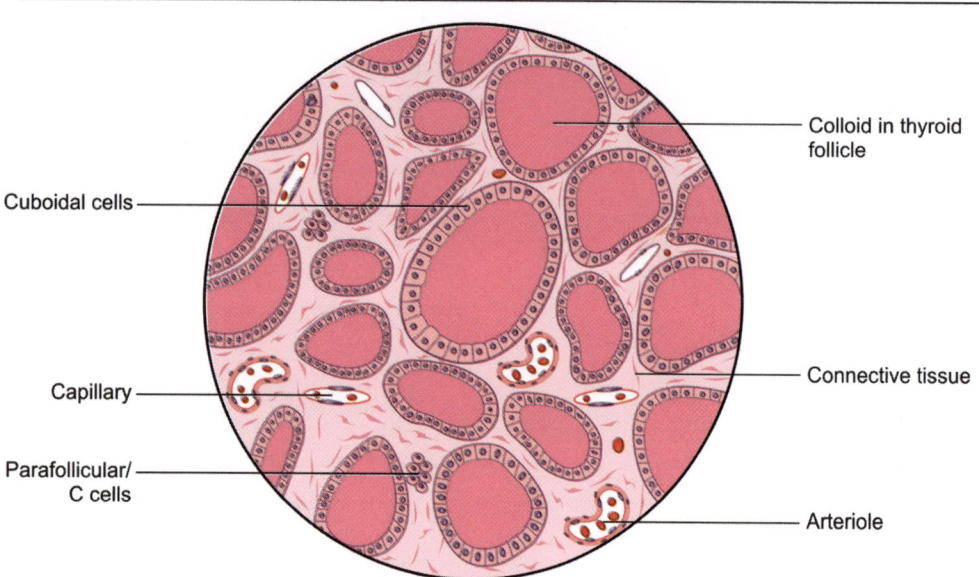

Cuboidal cells

Capillary

Parafollicular/
C cells

Colloid in thyroid
follicle

Connective tissue

Arteriole

Thyroid gland. Stain: Haematoxylin-eosin, 100X

PARATHYROID GLAND

The parathyroid glands are two pairs of small, yellow-brown bodies intimately connected with the posterior aspect of the thyroid gland. The parenchyma consists of *principal cells* and *oxyphilic cells*.

_____

_____

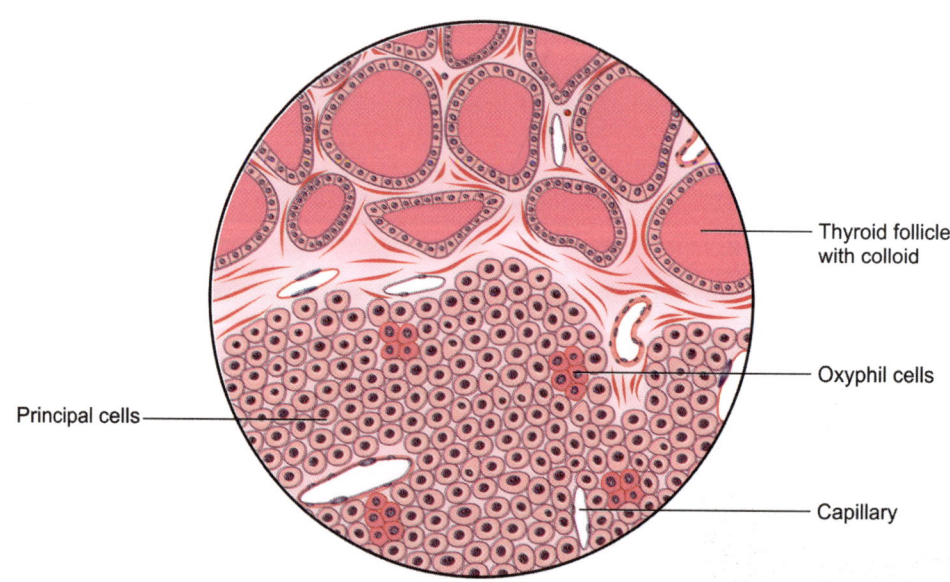

Principal cells

Thyroid follicle
with colloid

Oxyphil cells

Capillary

Thyroid and parathyroid glands. Stain: Haematoxylin-eosin, 100X

Thyroid Gland

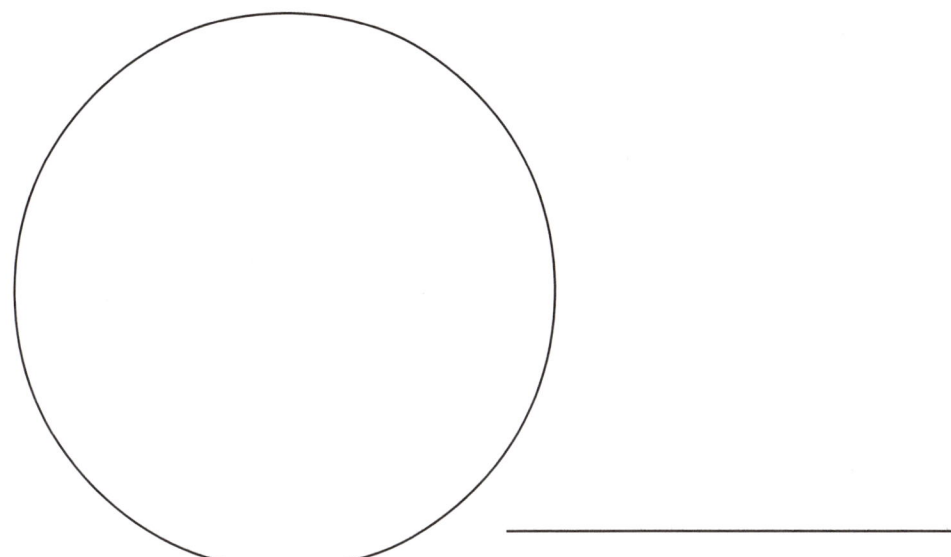

_____

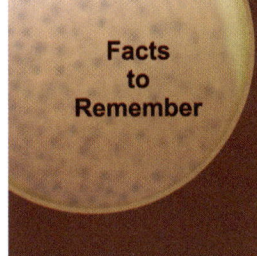

**Facts
to
Remember**

_____

_____

_____

Parathyroid Gland

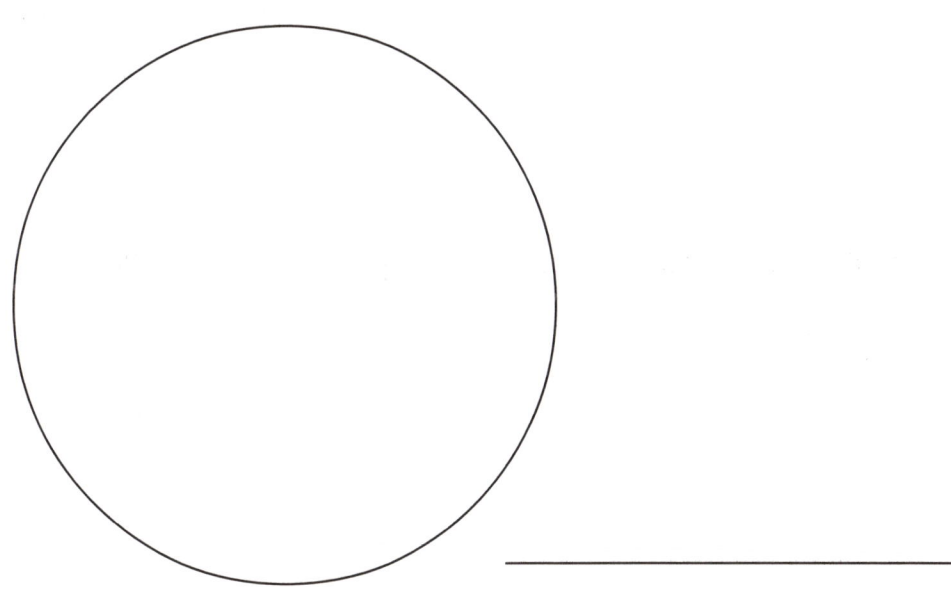

_____

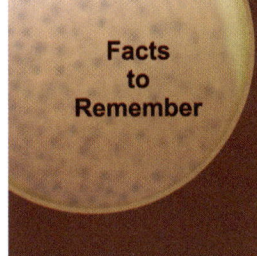

**Facts
to
Remember**

_____

_____

_____

SUPRARENAL OR ADRENAL GLAND

The paired suprarenal or adrenal glands are flattened glands, at the cranial pole of each kidney. Each gland is comprised of outer yellow cortex surrounding the inner dark brown medulla.

Cortex

_____

_____

_____

_____

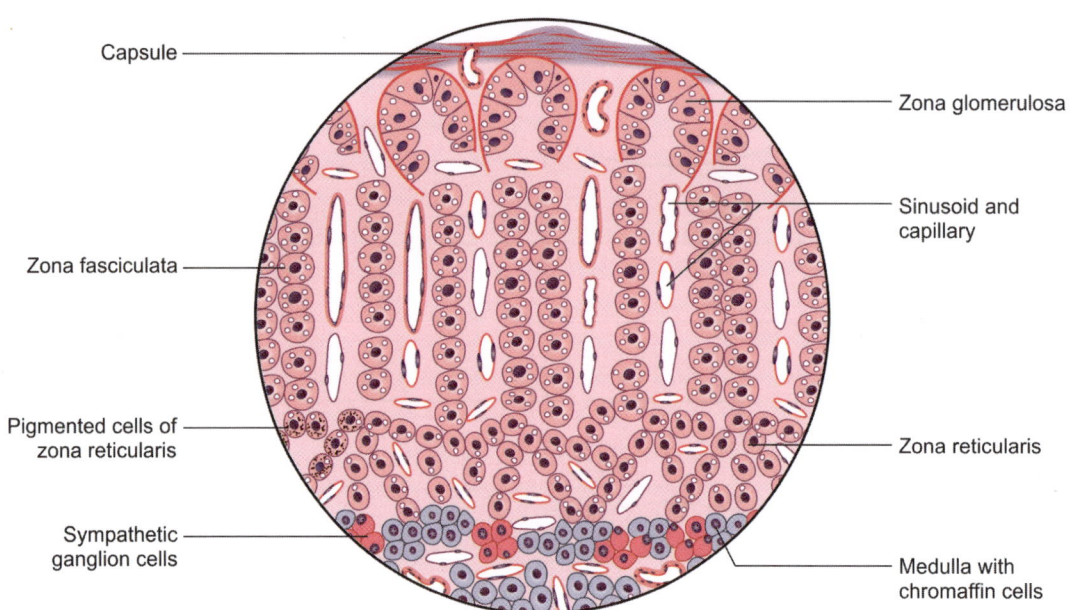

Capsule

Zona fasciculata

Pigmented cells of zona reticularis

Sympathetic ganglion cells

Zona glomerulosa

Sinusoid and capillary

Zona reticularis

Medulla with chromaffin cells

Suprarenal gland. Stain: Haematoxylin-eosin, 400X

Magnified View of the Zones and Medulla

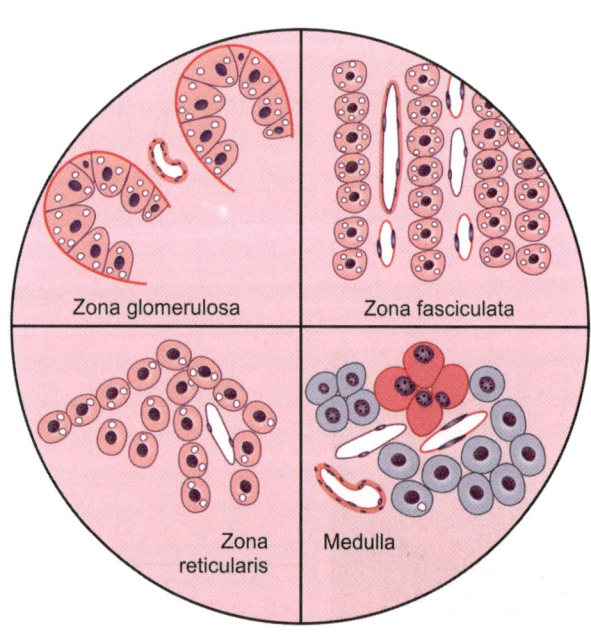

Zona glomerulosa

Zona fasciculata

Zona reticularis

Medulla

Suprarenal or Adrenal Gland

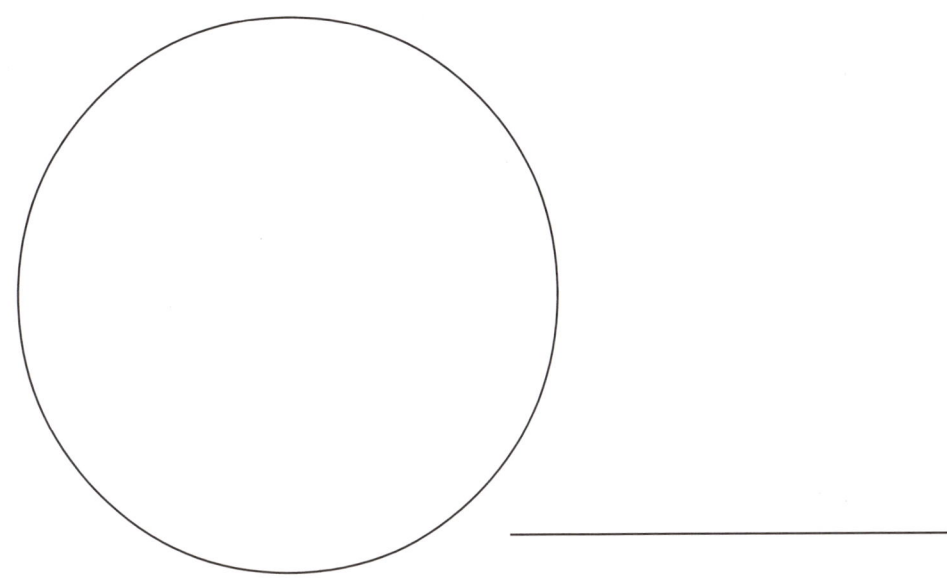

_____

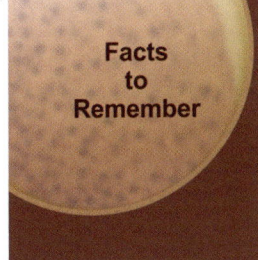

**Facts
to
Remember**

_____

_____

_____

Magnified View of the Zones and Medulla

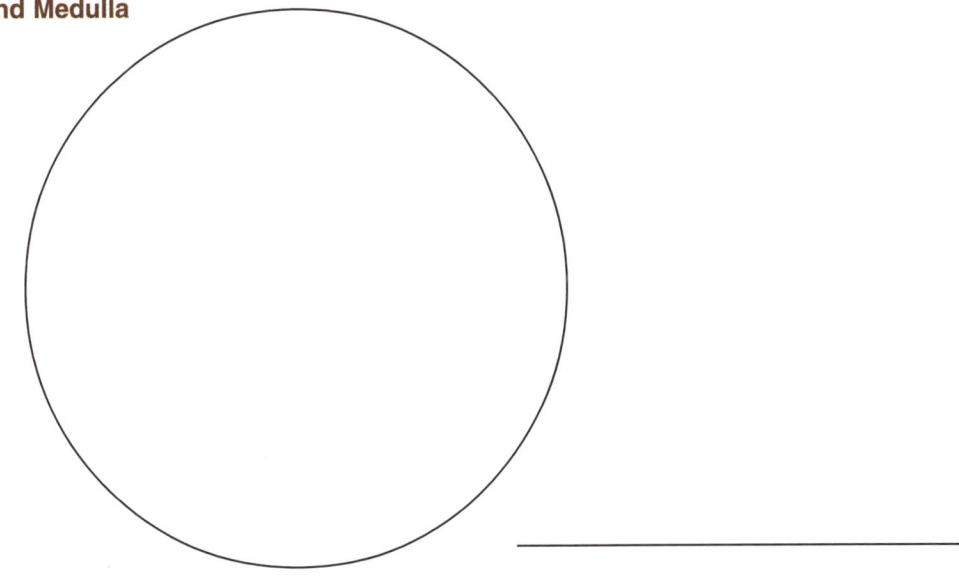

_____

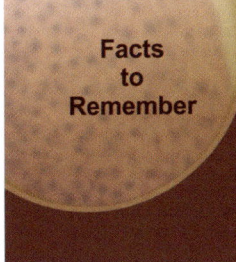

**Facts
to
Remember**

_____

_____

_____

ADDITIONAL FIGURES/NOTES

ADDITIONAL FIGURES/NOTES

19. Organs of Special Senses

OLFACTORY EPITHELIUM

The receptors of the sense of smell are located in the olfactory epithelium of nasal cavity. The epithelium is of tall *pseudostratified columnar* variety. Other layers are: _____

_____

_____

_____

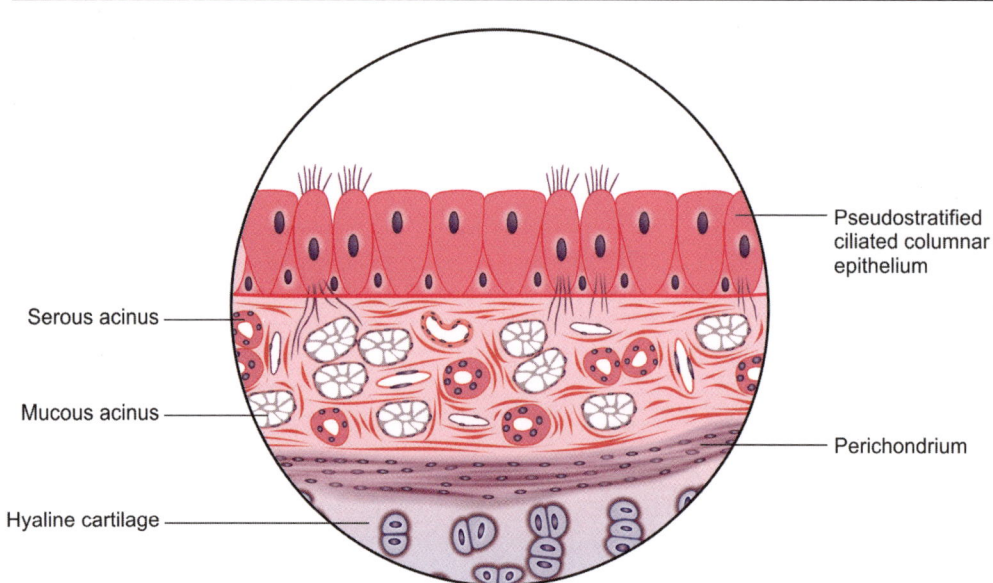

Layers of olfactory region. Stain: Haematoxylin-eosin, 400X

TONGUE

In the anterior two-thirds on the dorsal surface of tongue, the underlying corium consists of collagen and elastic fibres which project upwards forming *papillae*. Three types of papillae are present: The *filiform*, the *fungiform* and the *circumvallate*. The figure shows filiform and fungiform papillae.

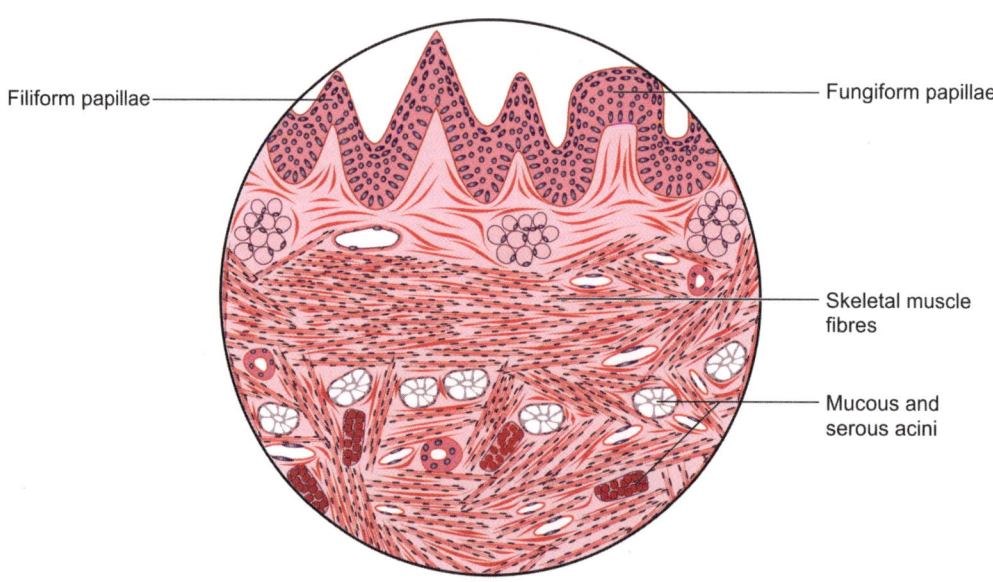

Anterier part of tongue with papillae. Stain: Haematoxylin-eosin, 100X

Olfactory Epithelium

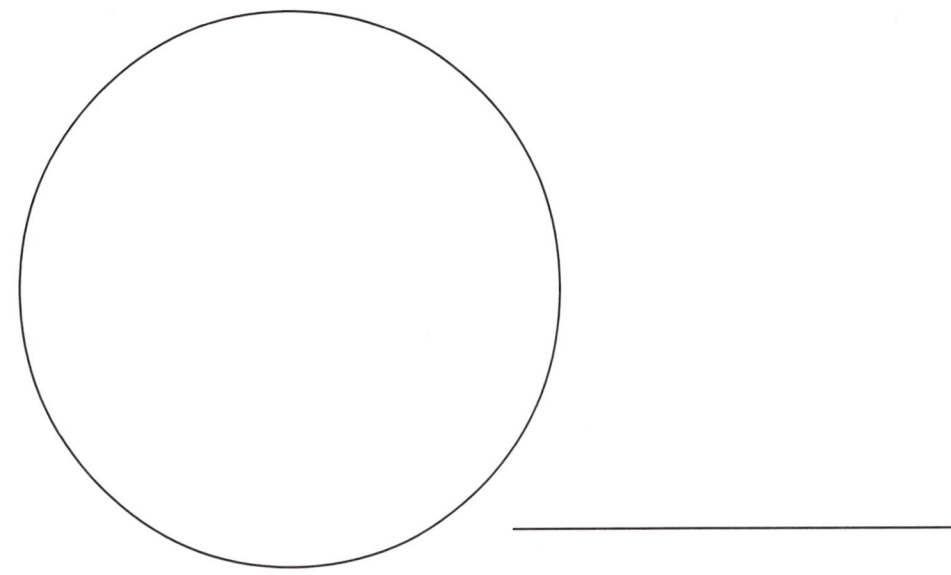

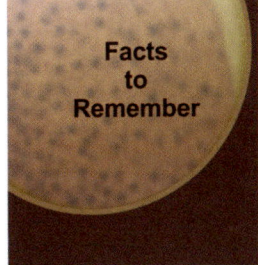

Facts
to
Remember

Tongue

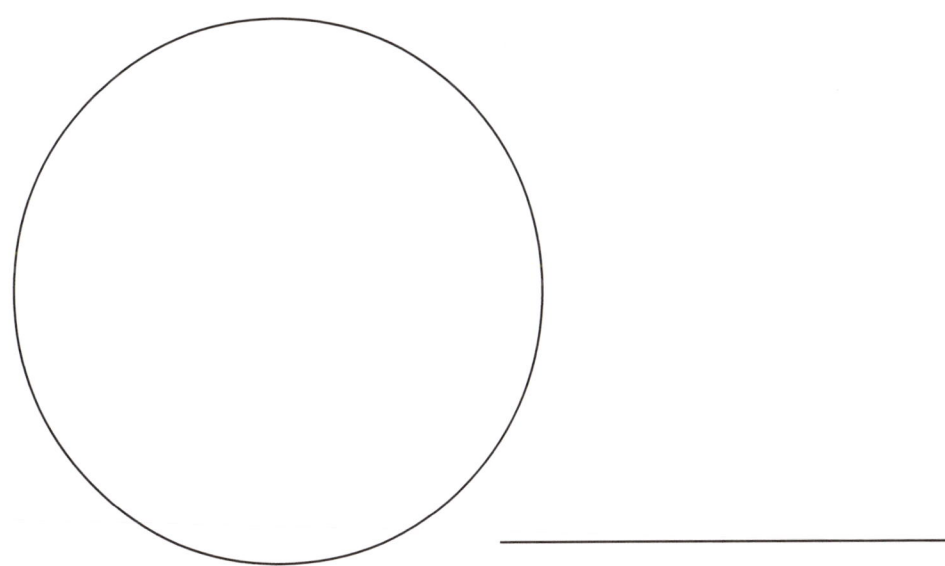

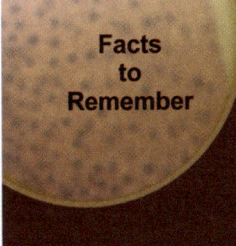

Facts
to
Remember

Circumvallate Papillae

The *circumvallate papillae* are bigger than the other two types of papillae and lie just anterior to the junction of the anterior two-thirds and the posterior one-third of the tongue. These comprise _____

_____

_____

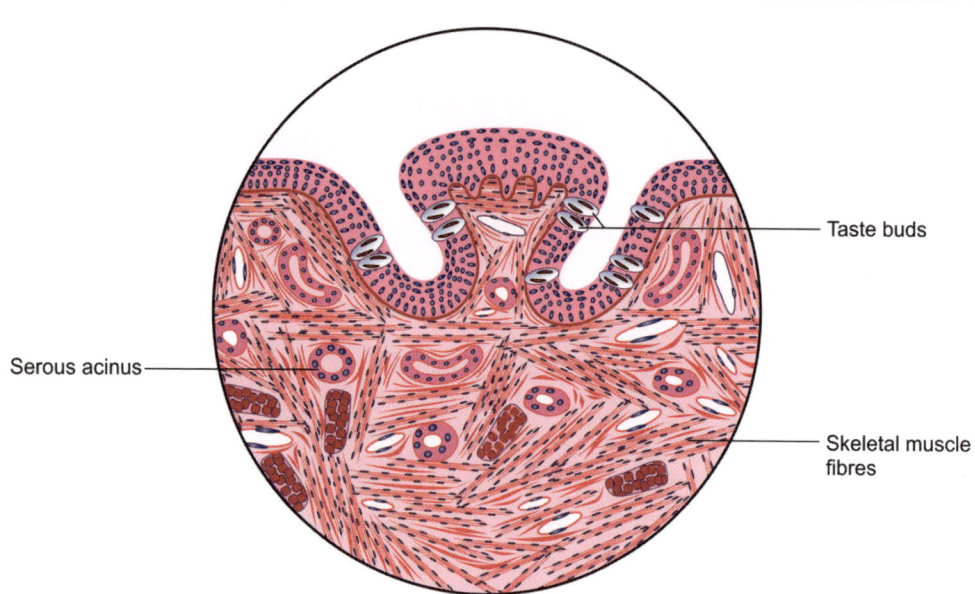

Circumvallate papilla. Stain: Haematoxylin-eosin, 100X

Taste Buds

The taste buds are seen mostly on the lateral sides of the circumvallate papillae. Taste buds are barrel-shaped structures, and comprising of the *supporting* or *sustentacular cells* and *neuroepithelial* or *gustatory cells:*

_____

_____

_____

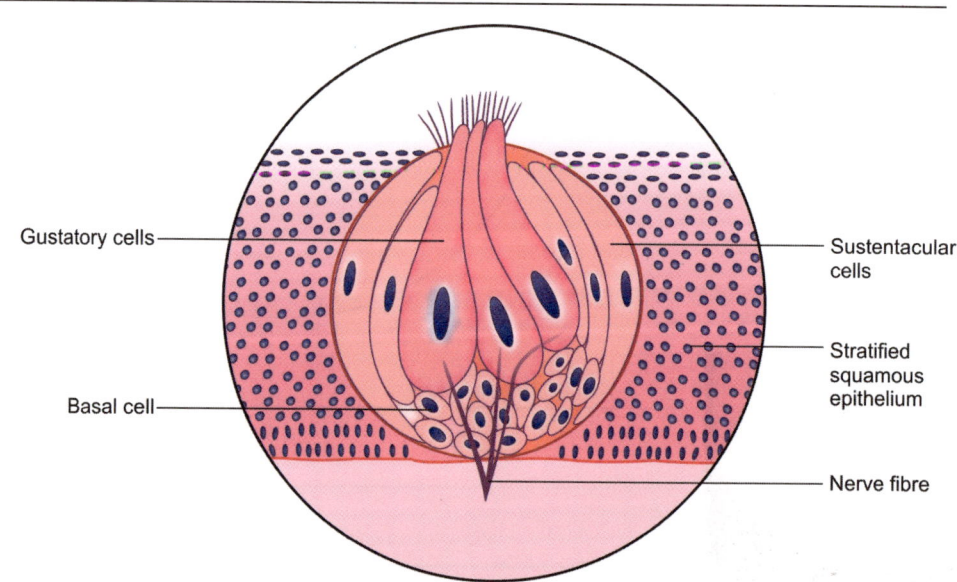

Taste bud. Stain: Haematoxylin-eosin, 400X

Circumvallate Papillae

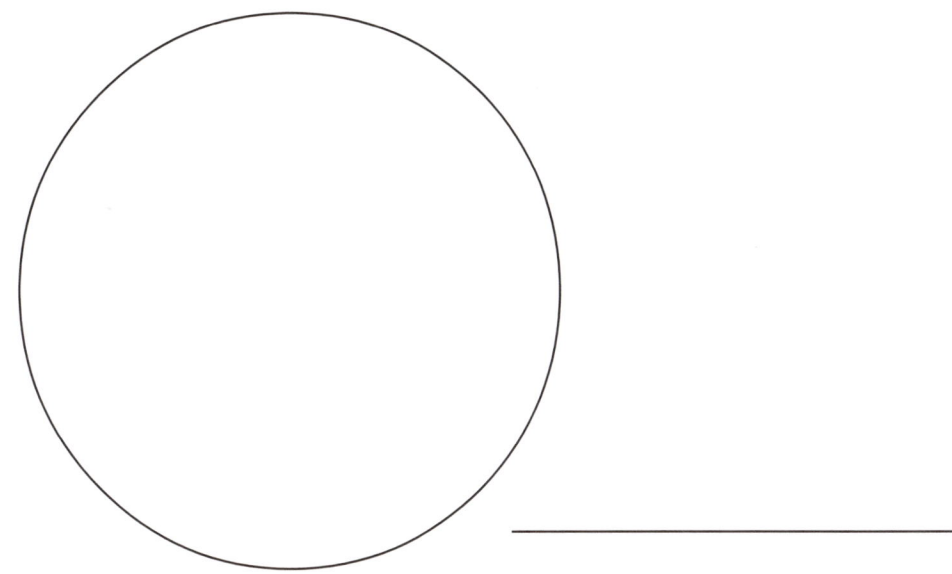

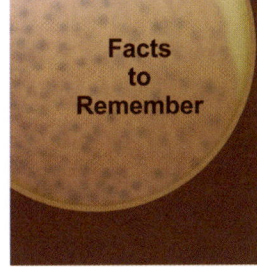

Facts
to
Remember

Taste Buds

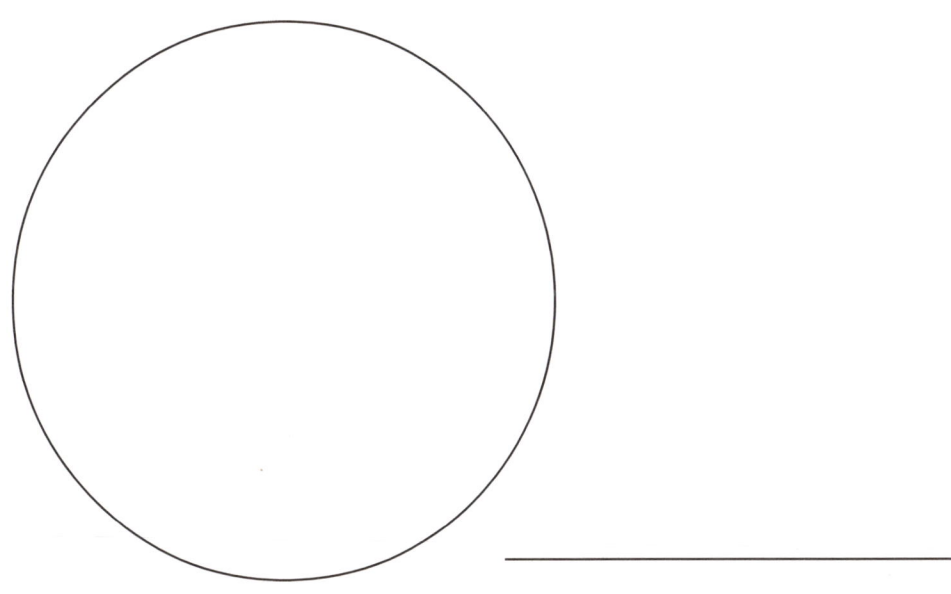

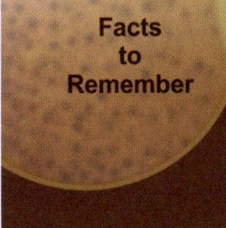

Facts
to
Remember

STRUCTURE OF THE EYEBALL

Cornea

_____

_____

_____

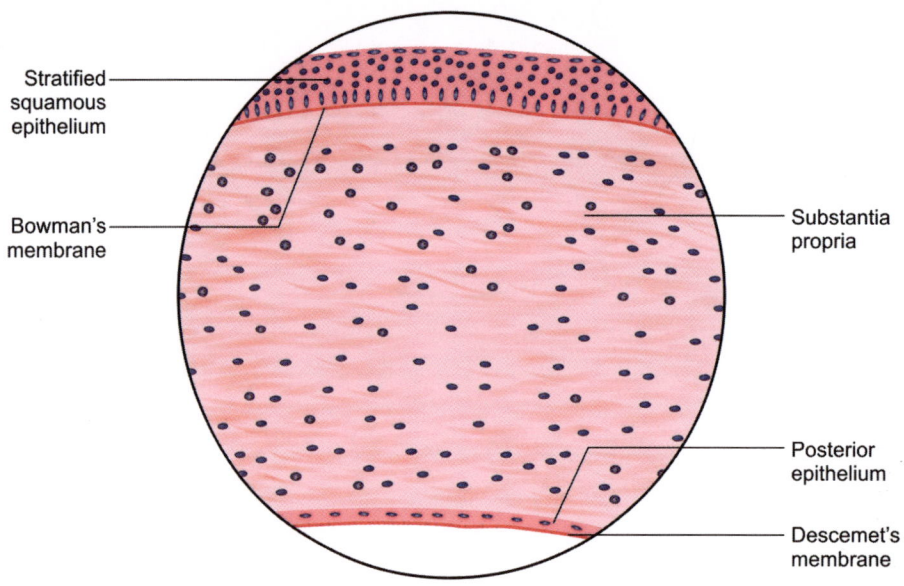

Cornea. Stain: Haematoxylin-eosin, 100X

Sclera and Choroid

_____

_____

_____

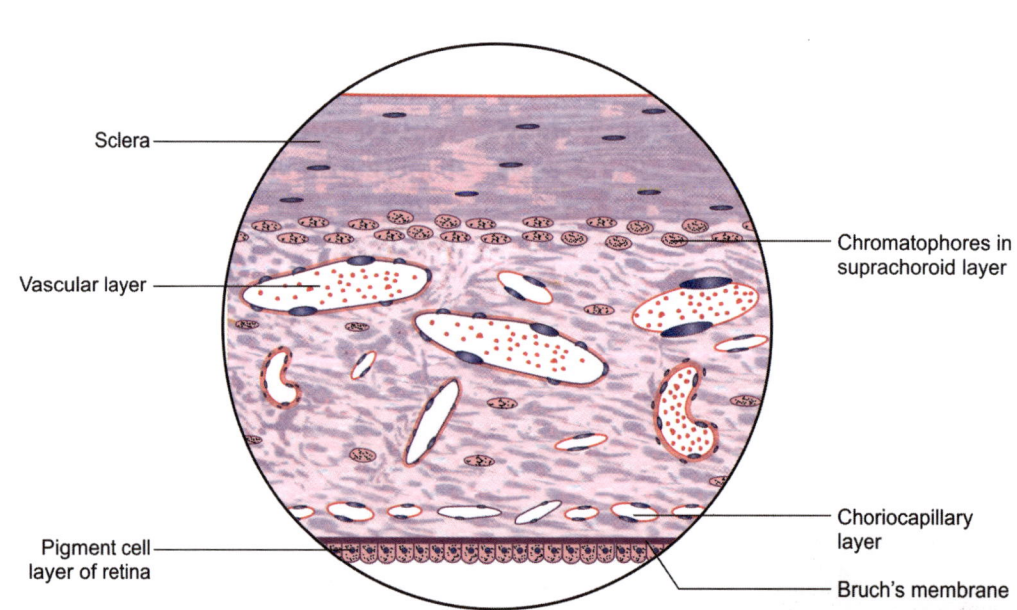

Sclera and choroid. Stain: Haematoxylin-eosin, 100X

Cornea

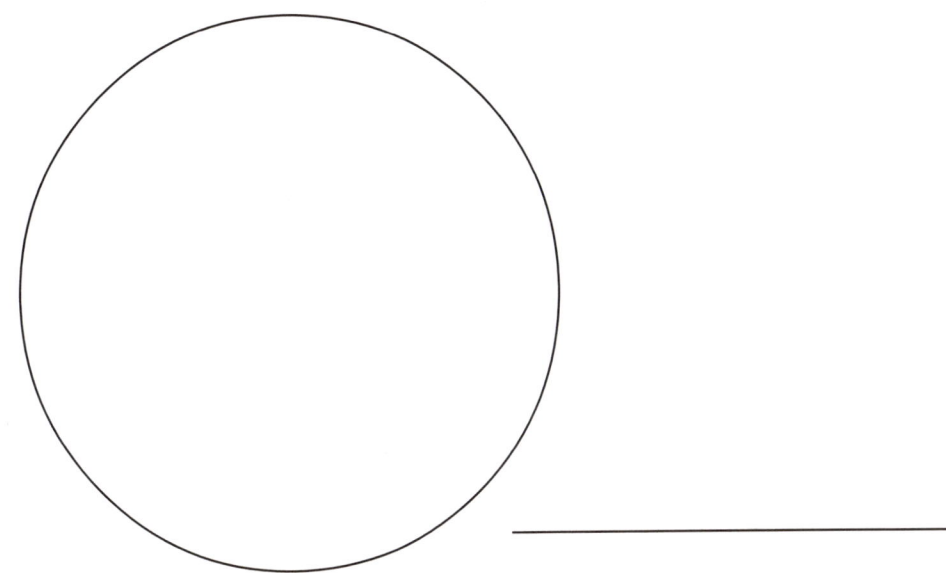

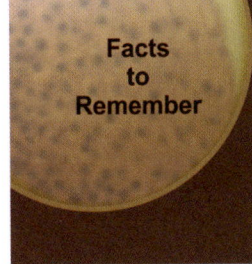

Facts
to
Remember

Sclera and Choroid

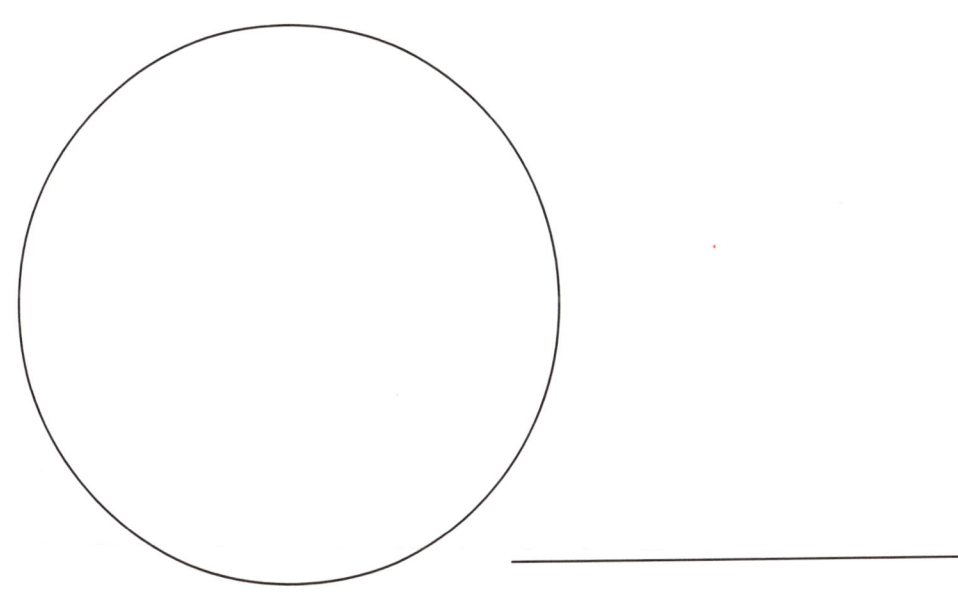

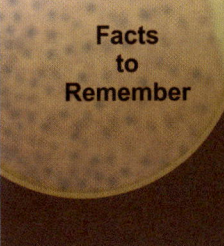

Facts
to
Remember

RETINA

Retina comprises ten parallel layers. Starting from the outer layers, these are:

1. _____

_____

2. _____

_____

3. _____

4. _____

_____

5. _____

_____

6. _____

_____

7. _____

_____

8. _____

_____

9. _____

_____

10. _____

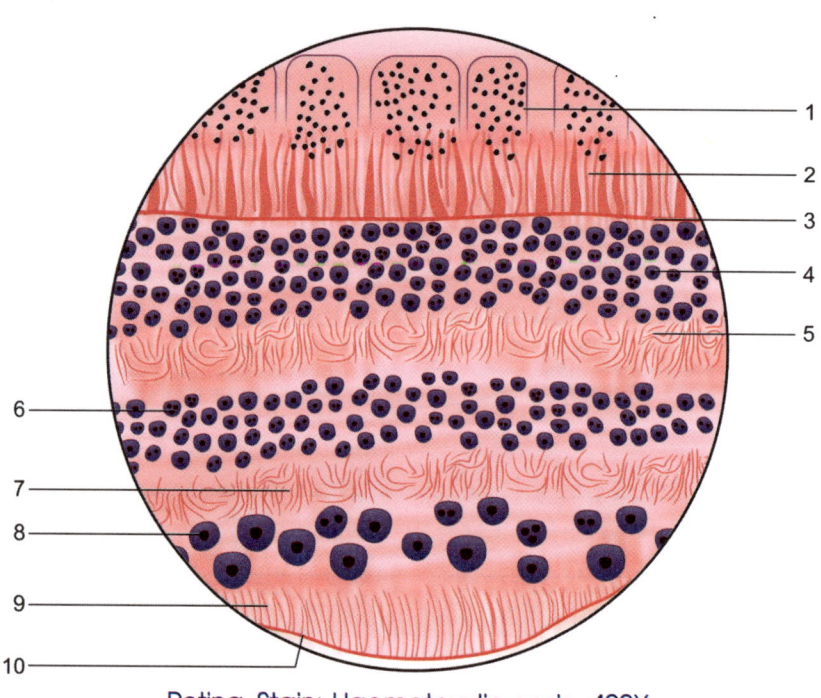

Retina. Stain: Haematoxylin-eosin, 400X

Retina

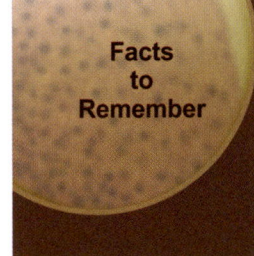

Facts to Remember

INTERNAL EAR

The internal ear is called labyrinth because of its complex structure. It is composed of a series of fluid-filled sacs and tubules suspended in cavities of corresponding form in the petrous part of the temporal bone.

There are two major cavities in the bony labyrinth—the vestibule which houses the saccule and the utricle of the membranous labyrinth. Anteromedial to it is the spirally coiled cochlea which contains the organ of Corti. The various cells of cochlea are: _____

_____

_____

_____

_____

_____

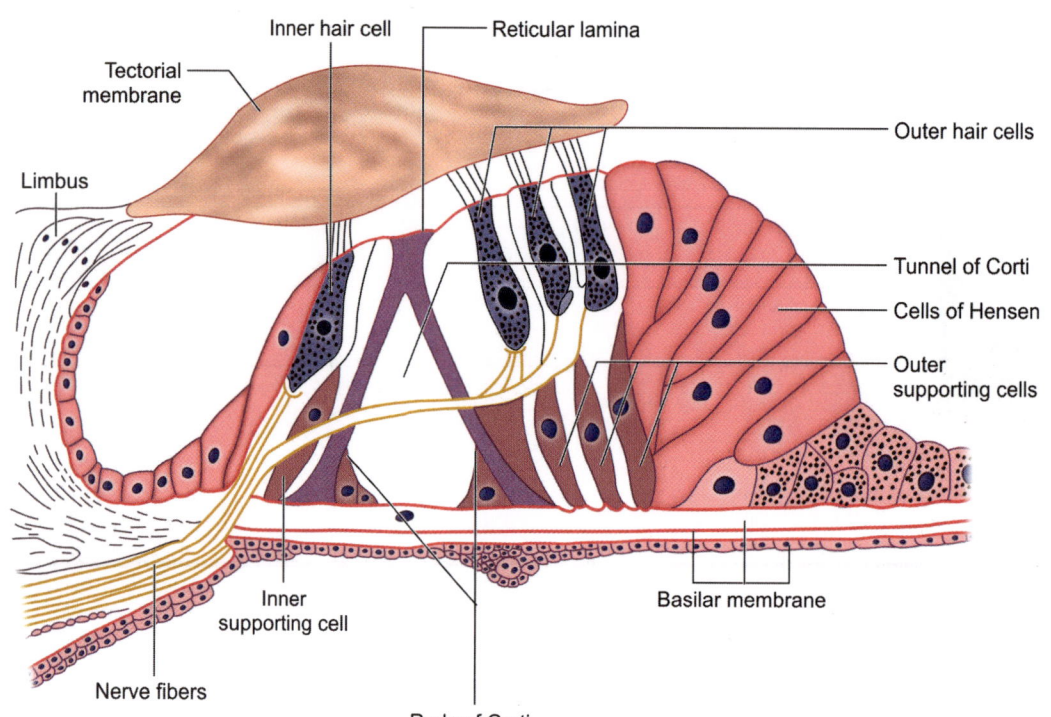

Part of the internal ear. Stain: Haematoxylin-eosin, 100X

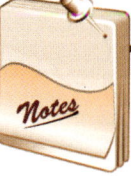

Internal Ear

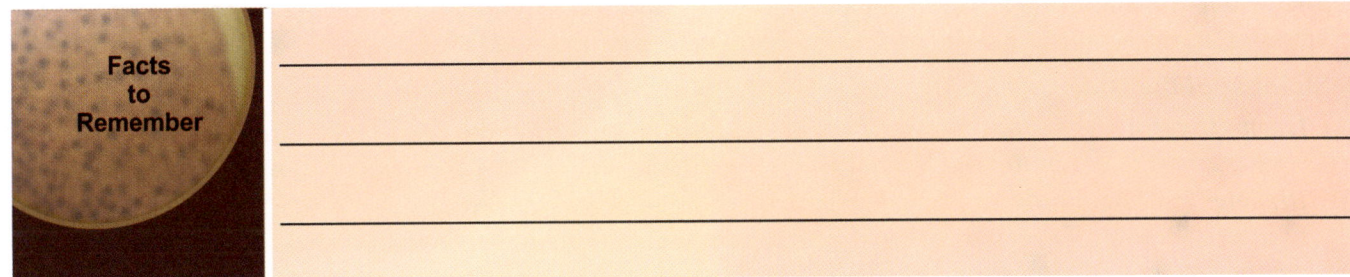

Facts to Remember

20. Staining: Haematoxylin-Eosin and Key to Identification of Histological Slides

STAINING: HAEMATOXYLIN-EOSIN

Requirements for Staining

Ehrlich's haematoxylin stain tested for five to seven minutes; water soluble eosin stain tested for half to one minute, Coplin jars containing xylol, absolute alcohol, 90 per cent alcohol, 70 per cent alcohol, 1 per cent acid alcohol, Canada balsam, slide rack, burner, coverslips, tap water, and blotting paper.

Procedure

Before proceeding with staining, the side of the tissue on the slide should be determined. The steps are as follows:

1. Removal of paraffin

i. Warm the slide on the reverse side of the tissue on a burner in order to melt the paraffin completely. The time varies according to the weather. Care should be taken not to burn the tissue.

ii. Dip the slide in xylol for 2–3 minutes to remove the paraffin.

2. Hydration of tissue

Dip the slide in descending series of alcohol, i.e. absolute alcohol, 90 per cent alcohol, 70 per cent alcohol and water for one minute each respectively. This procedure hydrates the tissue so that it is ready for staining with haematoxylin and eosin which are water soluble stains.

3. Staining of the slide

i. *Haematoxylin stain:* Place the slide on the slide-rack and cover the tissue with drops of haematoxylin stain for five to seven minutes. It stains the nucleus as well as the cytoplasm of the tissue.

Blueing: The haematoxylin stained slide is placed in a beaker of running tap water (alkaline pH) for ten to fifteen minutes. During this time the nucleus retains the stain whereas the stain is washed off from the cytoplasm. The differentiation of the cells is checked under low power of the microscope. If the tissue is seen to be overstained with haematoxylin, the slide is dipped in 1 per cent acid alcohol and then in water to remove the excess of stain.

ii. *Eosin stain:* Stain the tissue with a few drops of water soluble eosin solution for half to one minute and wash the slide with water. If the tissue gets overstained, the slide should be washed with running water till excess of stain is removed.

4. Dehydration of tissue

The slide is passed through the ascending grades of alcohol, i.e. 70 per cent, 90 per cent and absolute alcohol for one minute each. Finally it is dipped in xylol (clearing agent) to get rid of the alcohol. The section is blotted for mounting.

5. Mounting the slide

One drop of Canada balsam is put on the slide. A clean cover slip is gradually lowered on it so that air bubbles do not enter between the tissue and the coverslip.

Precautions

1. The slide should never be allowed to get dry.
2. If the tissue is overstained with haematoxylin, it should be treated with 1 per cent acid alcohol and then water.
3. In case of overstaining of tissue with eosin, the slide should be washed with water to remove excess of stain.

4. Cover slip should be gradually lowered on the slide in order to prevent entry of air bubbles.

5. During the process of staining care should be taken to avoid the tissue being washed off from the slide.

6. The slide should be examined under the microscope for proper differentiation.

KEY TO IDENTIFICATION OF HISTOLOGICAL SLIDES

See the Slide with Naked Eye

The slide may be

A. Tubular

B. Non-tubular structure/solid tissues

A. Tubular Structures

See the epithelium which will help in identification

1. **Simple squamous—may be artery/vein**

   Abundance of elastic fibres in tunica media—*elastic artery*

   Abundance of smooth muscle fibres in tunica media—*muscular artery*

   Small lumen with 2–3 layers of smooth muscle fibres—*arteriole*

   Big lumen, thick tunica adventitia with collagen fibres—*venule/vein*

2. **(i) Columnar epithelium and presence of muscularis mucosae**

   a. All cells looking alike with absence of goblet cells and epithelium invaginating to form glands—*stomach*

      • Fundus/body—3 layers of muscularis externa and long gastric glands with oxyntic cells

      • Pylorus—pyloric sphincter, mucous glands with long ducts

   b. Columnar epithelium evaginates to form villi, invaginates to form crypts and goblet cells present—*small intestine*

      • Duodenum—Brunner's (mucous) glands

      • Jejunum—no Brunner's glands, no Peyer's patches

      • Ileum—Peyer's patches

   c. Columnar epithelium invaginates to form lots of crypts, goblet cells preponderant—*colon*

      A few small crypts, lymphoid tissue abundant small lumen—*vermiform appendix*

   (ii) Columnar epithelium with absence of muscularis mucosae:

   a. With brush border and thin muscular coat—*gall bladder*.

   b. Columnar epithelium with simple glands and abundant smooth muscle fibres with arterioles—*uterus*

      • Simple gland—proliferative phase of endometrium.

      • Tortuous gland—progestational phase

      • Only basal part of gland with blood in lumen—menstrual phase of endometrium.

   c. Columnar ciliated epithelium thrown into folds with thin muscle layer—*fallopian tube*

3. **Pseudostratified ciliated columnar epithelium:**

   i. With a single large piece of hyaline cartilage and glands—*trachea*

   ii. With small pieces of cartilages and alveoli—*intrapulmonary bronchus*

   iii. With *no* cartilage, lumen surrounded by thick smooth muscle. Whole tissue seen under low power—*vas deferens*

   iv. Number of cut sections of tubules, surrounded by smooth muscle fibres—*epididymis*

   v. Mucous membrane showing cut section of folds, wall is thin—*seminal vesicle*

4. Stratified squamous non-keratinised epithelium: With muscularis mucosae—*oesophagus*
Same epithelium with no muscularis mucosae—*vagina*

5. Transitional epithelium: Star shaped lumen, whole slide is seen under low power—*ureter*
Same epithelium, big lumen with irregular arrangement of fibres—*urinary bladder*

B. No Lumen Seen/Solid Structure

1. Dark areas—*lymphoid tissue*
  i. Lymph nodules at the periphery and lymphatic cords in centre—*lymph node*
 ii. Lymph nodules all over with arteriole and red blood cell in between—*spleen*
iii. Lobulated lymphatic organ with epithelial cells around a hyaline mass—*thymus*
 iv. Lymph nodules lined by stratified squamous non-keratinised epithelium—*palatine tonsil*

2. Glands
  i. Well defined cells around a central vein and porta hepatis with 3 tubular structures—*liver*

 ii. **Salivary glands and pancreas**
      a. Serous acini and ducts—*parotid*
      b. Mucous acini, demilunes and ducts—*sublingual*
      c. Both serous and mucous acini with demilunes—*submandibular*
      d. Serous acini and light coloured islets of Langerhans' seen—*pancreas*

iii. **Endocrine glands**
      a. Lots of pink cells and blue cells in one area. Axons in another area—*hypophysis cerebri*
      b. Follicles lined by cuboidal to columnar cells with colloid in lumen—*thyroid*
      c. Polygonal cells in abundance with a few oxyphil cells. Thyroid follicles may also be seen— *parathyroid*
      d. Cells arranged in three zones with different arrangements of cells. The central part contains polygonal cells and ganglion cells—*suprarenal*

 iv. **Mammary gland/prostate**
      a. Ducts with intra and interlobular connective tissue and fibrofatty tissue—*resting mammary gland*
      b. Round/oval acini lined by columnar cells, a few ducts seen. Connective tissue seems minimal— *lactating mammary gland*
      c. Large irregular acini may contain corpora amylacea, urethra may be seen. Fibrous tissue and smooth muscle fibres seen—*prostate gland*

  v. **Parenchymatous organs**
      a. *Kidney:* Glomeruli, tubules and collecting ducts
      b. *Ovary:* Lots of follicles of varying size and shape
      c. *Testis:* Seminiferous tubules lined by stratified epithelium. In between are cells of Leydig.
      d. *Penis:* 3 rounded bodies— two corpra cavernosa and one corpus spongiosum

 vi. **Special senses**
      a. *Skin:* Epidermis with several layers of cells and appendages
      b. *Tongue:* Stratified squamous epithelium with papillae. Circumvallate papilla with taste buds.
      c. *Nasal mucous membrane:* Pseudostratified ciliated columnar with bipolar neurons
      d. *Cornea:* Stratified squamous non-keratinised epithelium, no papillae, substantia propria seen
      e. *Retina:* 3 layers of neurons and intervening nerve fibres
      f. *Organ of Corti:* Scala vestibuli and scala tympani and one scala media with rods of Corti and tectorial membrane

vii. Nervous tissue

    a. *Spinal cord*

        i. Grey matter

        ii. White matter

    b. *Ganglia*

        i. Autonomic ganglia

        ii. Spinal ganglia

    c. *Cerebellum*

    d. *Cerebrum*

viii. General histological slides

    a. *Loose connective tissue*

        i. Areolar tissue: Collagen fibre bundles, a few elastic fibres and cells

        ii. Adipose tissue: Fat cells and collagen fibres

        iii. Reticular tissue: Small thin curved fibres stained by silver stains

        iv. Myxomatous tissue

    b. *Dense connective tissue:* Collagen fibre bundles with fibroblasts

    c. *Cartilage:*

      Hyaline: Chondrocytes in cell nests, fibres not visible

      Elastic: Single chondrocytes with elastic fibres

      Fibro: Thick bundles of collagen fibres with a few chondrocytes

    d. *Bone:* Compact with haversian lamellae

          Cancellous with trabeculae and big marrow spaces

    e. *Muscles:* Striated—with striations and multiple peripheral nuclei

          Smooth—with spindle shaped cells and central single nucleus

          Cardiac—short branching fibres with central nucleus and intercalated discs

ix. Others

    a. *Umbilical cord:* With three vessels, two arteries and one vein. Outer covering is amnion.

    b. *Placenta:* Oval chorionic villi with capillaries and RBC in between villi

    c. *Cervix:* Inner part lined by columnar epithelim and outer part lined by stratified squamous non-keratinising epithelium.

ADDITIONAL FIGURES/NOTES

Reader's Note